Meike Wiedemann || Kirsten Segler

Neurofeedback

KIRSTEN SEGLER || MEIKE WIEDEMANN

NEUROFEEDBACK

A gentle therapy to help the brain help itself

Translation: Deirdre Winter and Elizabeth Hamilton

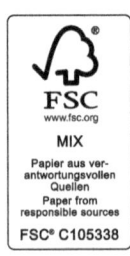
Dr. rer. nat. **Meike Weidemann** is a neurobiologist and therapist with her own practice in Stuttgart, Germany. She has been working with neurofeedback for nearly 30 years and is actively engaged in advancing ILF, in particular, through research projects and training.

Kirsten Segler is also a biologist. However, after gaining her degree she turned to journalism. She writes for magazines such as Men's Health and Brigitte and is also the author of books on the subjects of health, diet and nature.

1. Edition 2024
Copyright © 2024 Meike Wiedemann, Kirsten Segler
Translation:
Deirdre Winter, B.A. Hons. (Interpreting and Translating), Dipl. Psych.
www.transwinter.de
Elizabeth Hamilton, B.A. Hons. (German), M.Phil (German), Dip Trans (German and French)
Coverdesign: Weiss Werkstatt Munich
Illustrations: Stefan Dangl, Munich
Photos: page 58 Edith Schneider, page 63 EEGinfo.ch
Satz, Herstellung und Verlag: BoD – Books on Demand, Norderstedt
ISBN 978-3-7583-7509-5

This book is also available as an E-Book.

CONTENTS

You don't need to know anything about "the little gray cells" to be helped by neurofeedback.
But if you are interested, in this part of the book you can find out more about how the brain makes it possible for us to experience the present, how it produces memories and shapes our dreams of the future.

In discussions about neurofeedback you often find three fundamentally different approaches lumped together, which do, however, need to be clearly distinguished from one another. Their most important common feature is that to clients they all seem easy and fun.

Here you will find out how neurofeedback therapy can be helpful in twelve different disorders and their various symptoms. Common to all these problems is the fact that the healthy balance between the brain's fundamental excitability and its capacity to regulate itself has been lost.

WHAT IS NEUROFEEDBACK?

When I caught the neurofeedback bug I was about to become a laboratory assistant in the pharmaceutical industry. I was just completing my degree in neurobiology and was looking through the most recent studies on migraine in preparation for my diploma thesis. I was particularly interested in the question as to how the brain manages to regulate and control its excitability and the extent to which excitation develops and spreads. One of the greatest challenges of the nervous system is to fine-tune stimulating and inhibiting impulses – we might think of this as stepping on the gas or putting on the brakes – so that we are able to do what we have to do in the best possible way. If this doesn't go well, a number of very different of symptoms can result, migraine being just one example among many.

With all my neurobiological knowledge about the structure of the brain and the important role of neurotransmitters, my initial impulse was to look for the solution in chemical substances – i.e. active pharmacological ingredients that might be able to help the brain to better manage its excitation levels. However, in the course of my searches I came across the idea of neurofeedback and I was immediately electrified. It was claimed that patients could use devices to train themselves to better regulate their brains, and that by so doing they could learn to create a healthy balance in the excitability of their nervous system and thus prevent attacks of migraine or epilepsy. If that is possible, I thought, what else might the brain be able to learn to do with if it was supported by the right feedback signals? I couldn't wait to find out more about this! From then on I was infected by enthusiasm for neurofeedback, and, as it turned out, it was quite a serious infection. Today I am still in the thrall of this kind of therapy – in fact my fascination grows from day to day.

That all happened a good 20 years ago, and the world was quite different then. Those were the early days of the internet, for example, and nobody could envisage how radically that was going to change our lives. In those days, the genome was viewed as an immutable template for all our bodily functions, whereas today we know that genes are not simply something that we possess, but that they can be switched on and off depending on the environmental conditions the organism has to contend with. Moreover, the fact that the brain has the capacity to develop was not so widely known. The dogma at that time was that adults cannot form new nerve cells and it was therefore thought that after a certain age it is impossible to make any decisive changes to the way the brain is organized. I'm sure you know the saying "You can't teach an old dog new tricks." Nothing could be further from the truth.

In fact the brain can be modified well into old age. This capacity is known as neuroplasticity. We can see how pronounced it is if we look at stroke patients. The more they exercise the more likely it is that the tasks previously performed by the damaged areas of the brain will be taken over by other areas. Some experiments conducted by the American neurophysiologist Paul Bach-Y-Rita, a pioneer in research into neuroplasticity, are also most impressive. He managed to render sensory impressions experienceable in new ways. For example, he created apparatuses that transform pictures taken by a camera into electrical impulses and transfer them to a metal plate so that they can be perceived by blind people by means of their tongues. The harder blind people practice, the better they can "see" again. Their brain learns to turn the signals they have felt into pictures.

Today we know that in the same way that muscles get stronger if we use them a lot and place demands on them, the brain can also expand its capacities through exercising. It always adjusts to what the situation demands. But it is also lazy and tries to do what it has to do with the minimum of effort. In other words, it loves routine and likes best to follow well-worn paths – even if these are rather rocky. However, if it has to do something differently from before it has to be coaxed out of its complacency. One of the most powerful ways to do this is to evoke curiosity, enthusiasm and fun – i.e. states in which we are relaxed, but at the same time cheerful and outward-looking. If we had a kind of rev counter for the brain on our heads it would show that it is in these states that it is at an optimal level of excitation, with the revs being neither too low nor too high.

On a bell-shaped curve that I like to draw for my clients, this state is represented by the plateau at the top of the arc. This is where people are particularly productive because this is the arousal level that provides them with the most possible ways to act and react and will even make them capable of trying out completely new strategies. Thus it becomes more likely that the brain will find a way to reach a desired goal. And "goal" here can also mean quite ordinary things like making friendly contact with someone, concentrating on a task and enjoying performing it or simply sitting in the sunshine enjoying having an ice-cream and taking real pleasure in it.

However, with many disorders of brain function the problem is precisely that people who are affected by them do not, or no longer, achieve this optimal level of activation, or only far too rarely. And this is where neurofeedback comes in. The training helps the brain to learn how it can more easily get out of states in which the revs are too high or too low and access the relaxed and open state at the top of the curve in the graph. This is a necessary requirement if the nervous system is to be able to structure itself differently, continue to develop and perhaps even continue to mature. However, this process takes place not so much during the practical therapy sessions as in the clients' normal daily lives. Being able to maintain an optimal level of neural arousal more frequently and for longer periods of time broadens the perception of clients' perception and also how they feel. They can try out new behaviors which will lead them to experience things differently from the way they did before. A child with ADHD, whose lack of impulse control used to get them into trouble everywhere, may experience for the very first time how they can join in with a group of children playing and feel accepted by the others on this happy afternoon. Pleasant experiences like this consolidate the new strategies, and nothing else is required. The brain structures itself anew through what it experiences.

I continue to be delighted by the fact that all of this can be achieved by a form of treatment that is so easy and effortless for the clients – they simply watch films or play on the computer. I am particularly pleased about how easy it is because many of them (and their families as well!) have had to struggle so much in the past.

I must also thank my doctoral supervisor Professor Wolfgang Hanke of the University of Hohenheim for enabling me to work with this wonderful method. At a time when feedback was still regarded as somewhat suspect, he was open-minded about my new passion and allowed me to pursue my own path in this direction. I am also particularly grateful to Sue and Siegfried Othmer in the USA, who developed the ILF neurofeedback that I work with. In my view, in the majority of cases it is this very modern branch of the neurofeedback method that gets the best results.

Many people are skeptical when they see the long list of indications for which neurofeedback claims to be effective (see Appendix). In fact you might easily get the impression that this method should be advertised as a cure-all. However, it is easy to explain why it can have such a positive effect on so many conditions. They all have one important thing in common – arousal in the nervous system is not regulated as well as it should be. Sometimes that is the underlying cause of the problem – as is almost always the case with migraine – and sometimes it is just part of the problem. With chronic back pain, for example, neurofeedback can help if the pain is triggered or exacerbated by excessive tension. However, if the root of the problem is structural damage, such as a fractured vertebra, brain training will usually be unsuccessful. It is also important to be aware that neurofeedback is often just one part of more comprehensive treatment and that it needs to be supplemented with coaching, psychotherapy, family counseling, massage or movement training.

And actually it is not neurofeedback that I am so passionate about anyway, but the brain – this infinitely fascinating organ that can deal with paradoxical demands simultaneously and allow us humans not only to experience the world passively but also even to create something completely new. The Othmers' way of viewing the brain has left its mark on me most. For them there is never anything wrong with it or anything that needs repair, nothing needs to be stimulated or blocked by medication. They are convinced that most dysfunctions are merely a sign that the nervous system lacks practice in this one particular area and that targeted training exercises can help it to acquire the capacities that it is missing. And that is how I see it too – and my clients would support me in this view again and again. It is always immensely satisfying to see how someone can liberate themselves from the restrictions of their illness by their own efforts and can begin to lead a more fulfilled life.

I hope this book will give many people with such conditions some useful suggestions and ideas to help them achieve this goal.

Dr Meike Wiedemann

I first came across neurofeedback when I was researching ADHD in adults, and I immediately succumbed to the fascination of this form of therapy. I have always been attracted to methods which train both the body and the mind and which promote a good response rather than intervening in the system by prescribing pills or doing surgery – even if this may initially appear easier.

If you agree with this view and are looking for a new way of treating a mental illness, a neurological disorder or other chronic problems, then neurofeedback could be the right thing for you. This book will give you an idea of whether you might like to try out this form of therapy for yourself or for your child or whether you might like to recommend it to someone in your family.

The first part of this book is devoted to the brain – it describes how this mysterious organ works and enables us to experience the world. In the second part you will be introduced to the three different forms of neuro-feedback. And finally, the third part deals with the main disturbances of brain function for which neurofeedback therapy offers good prospects of improvement (see Appendix for further symptoms and conditions). In Part Three we will give numerous examples from real cases to give you an idea of what the treatment is like and how the clients respond to it in practice. Naturally we have changed names and personal details so that they remain anonymous.

It would be wonderful if you might also have an encouraging story to tell as well.

Kirsten Segler

PART 1

The Brain and Nervous System

You don't in fact need to know anything about the brain in order to be able to benefit from neurofeedback. But perhaps you are one of those people who would like to have at least a rough idea of how the nervous system works so that you can more easily imagine how this treatment that seems so mysterious produces its effects. This part of the book gives you a brief description of how the brain operates — how it enables us to experience the present and how it evokes memories and shapes our dreams of the future.

The brain is not exactly pretty. You wouldn't, for instance, want to put it on a car sticker, like a heart, or use it as an icon in funny text messages, even as an abstract graphic image. Its gray and white surface is too pale and its convoluted folds and furrows too unruly. The brain of an adult human being weighs about 3.3 lbs and consists mainly of fat. Nature has gone to considerable lengths to protect it: not only does it pack the brain in a hard shell made of bone, it also provides us with a "blood-brain barrier" which acts as a strictly controlled boundary within the body's metabolic system. The "gray cells" between the ears are so precious that toxic substances must on no account reach them.

But how do these cells produce consciousness, thoughts, feelings and memories? You will learn more about this in the next few chapters, although in fact no-one has yet been able to completely solve this mystery. But one thing is certain: it is wrong to compare the brain to a computer, because not even the most advanced technical devices have the ability to create something genuinely new. If we need a comparison, then bread dough is perhaps somewhat less elegant, but a better analogy. In order to start rising, dough needs warmth and the right nourishment, it always yields to the hands that knead it, but it also develops on its own and adapts to its environment.

The brain in fact consists of just such interactions between external and internal forces. They continue to shape it into old age, always in such a way that it achieves the best possible fit with the given circumstances. If it receives only a few stimuli it simply develops the same nerve connections into wider and wider avenues. But if it is kept busy and challenged in a large number of inspiring ways, new pathways are constantly produced. It is not merely a question of what the outside world offers the brain objectively, but also of how it subjectively perceives these actualities. Is the glass half empty or half full? Is it better to cling to what we have and are familiar with, or to risk venturing into the unknown? Inner attitudes like this can be changed. Sometimes all we need to do in order to change is to come to a decision, but often we have to keep practicing hard, and sometimes we may even need the support of a coach or therapist.

It is worth expanding our comfort zone further and further because it is the many cross-connections that make the brain lively, creative and flexible. These connections are especially important when an area of the brain is damaged and other parts have to take over its tasks. It takes a lot of laborious effort to learn to walk again following a brain injury, but it often leads to success in the end. This is probably one of the most impressive examples of neuroplasticity, i.e. the malleability of the nervous system. Another is that since text messages sent from our phones have conquered the world, the region of the brain that is responsible for the movement of the thumbs has become appreciably larger, particularly in teenagers – because their thumbs have to be much more dexterous than they were in the previous generation.

Similarly, how you have treated the "dough" between your ears to date is reflected in how your brain performs. If you are not so happy with the result, what you need to do is change the conditions, experiment to find out what does you good – and "knead" your brain into the "shape" you want.

1. THE CEREBRUM

WELCOME TO THE EXECUTIVE SUITE!

Typically, a tour through the anatomy of the brain starts right at the top – in the cerebral cortex, which has multiple folds and is divided into two halves. This is because it is this part of the brain that most clearly distinguishes us human beings from other living organisms. It enables our species to make plans and to share them with other human beings, to invent stories and create things that are completely new.

The thinking center is behind the forehead

As shown in the next figure, each of the two halves of the cerebral cortex has four regions which are separated by deep grooves. Each of these regions is responsible for specific tasks. For example, the occipital lobes, which are mainly responsible for vision, lie at the back of the skull, while the temporal lobes, which are located at the side round the ears, take care of hearing and language comprehension (however, the latter function is usually located on the left side only). They are also involved in the regulation of the emotions and their effects on the body. The parietal lobes are situated at the back, under the crown, and are concerned with perception of the body, its orientation in space and intentionally executed movements. The brain functions that we refer to as "higher" functions, such as conscious thought processes and abstract ideas, arise in the frontal lobes, which are behind the forehead – in the very place we instinctively associate with these capacities.

The locations of the different regions of the brain

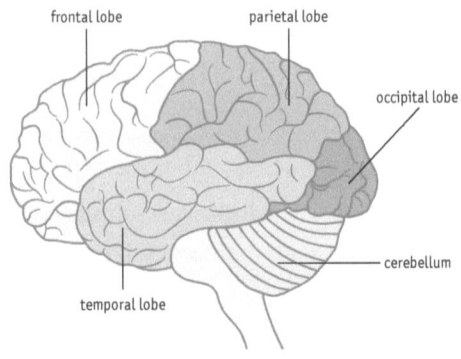

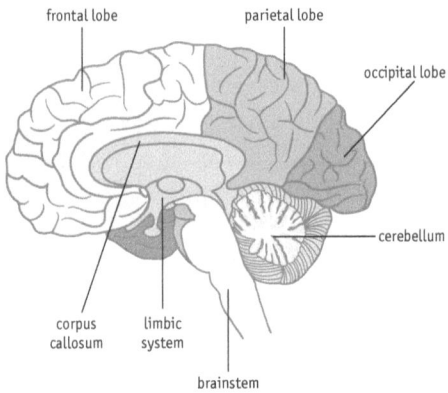

The two sides of the brain are connected by the corpus callosum, below which are most modules of the limbic system (which are only roughly sketched in this illustration).

One area of the brain, which is called the "prefrontal cortex", is decisive if we are to lead successful lives. It is the region most closely linked to ego consciousness, since it is where we consciously experience feelings and assess question, "What does this have to do with me?" It is here that events take on their own specific meanings. The prefrontal cortex also controls our ability to concentrate and our willpower. It ensures that we are not completely at the mercy of our impulses, but can postpone our responses in the service of a more important goal. For example, if we want to lose weight, we need a well-developed prefrontal cortex to enable us to refrain from eating too many cookies during a boring meeting. However, brain and behavior researchers now know that disciplined decisions use up a lot of energy, so we can make life easier for ourselves if we don't overtax our busy frontal lobe unnecessarily, and put the goodies out of sight.

Of all the brain regions, the prefrontal cortex takes the longest to fully develop in childhood. It doesn't "go online" at all until the age of about 18 to 24 months and doesn't become fully mature until long after puberty. This long developmental period makes it especially susceptible to disturbances. Many mental problems have to do with the fact that the prefrontal cortex is too weak, to put it simply. Fortunately in many cases it can still be trained and strengthened, even in adults. You will learn more about this later on in the book, since this is precisely where neurofeedback can help.

What can happen when a person has to do without this "impulse control center" is illustrated by the case of Phineas Gage. This man worked on the railroad in the 19th century and was injured in a gruesome accident in 1848. An explosion drove an iron bar through his cheek into his brain and destroyed his left prefrontal lobe. Amazingly he survived this injury, but he was never the same again. Whereas he had previously been a resolute and hard-working man, he now became a dissolute drunkard and was constantly after women. He was also no longer able to carry out his plans. But what happened to him provided science with some invaluable insights into how a person's personality is shaped by the body.

Nonidentical twins

Much of what we know about how the various tasks of the brain are distributed across the two halves (hemispheres) of the cortex has also been gained from observation of people suffering from severe illnesses. Many of these were patients with epilepsy in whom it became necessary to sever the connection between the two halves of the brain. This operation prevents seizures from spreading to the whole of the brain and they remain restricted to one half. However, it also prevents the active exchange of information across the corpus callosum, a thick bundle of "data cables" that consists of millions of nerve fibers. Normally the two halves of the brain work well together as a result of this constant communication, so that so long as we are healthy we hardly ever notice what is really going on "up there". Each hemisphere constructs a worldview of its own. The left side of the brain thinks in words (as mentioned above, this is where the capacity for language is located), sees things in an abstract and analytical way, is especially concerned with detail and has a sense of past and future. In contrast, the right half lives completely in the here-and-now, is more feeling-oriented, develops more imaginative ideas which, however, remain relatively vague, and processes impressions in a more global way. Its strength is its capacity to recognize patterns.

Put simply, the right side of the brain sees the woods, while the left side sees each individual tree. This teamwork between the two hemispheres makes it possible for the brain to avoid having to make compromises. Instead it can develop two completely opposing modes of perception and sets of capacities in parallel, and that to a very high degree. It can then combine these two extremes – the comprehensive, but relatively rough global view of the right hemisphere, which is influenced by emotions, and at the same time the more matter-of-fact, precise and detailed tunnel vision of the left hemisphere, which always focuses only on smaller segments.

> In some people – especially in those who are left-handed – the brain can also be organized somewhat differently from the way described above.

Even in healthy brains the two hemispheres do not function completely on an equal footing; usually the left hemisphere is more dominant. The neuroscientist Jill Bolte-Taylor gives an impressive description of what happens when the right hemisphere's way of viewing things suddenly pushes to the fore. One morning her left brain hemisphere became increasingly incapacitated, due to a burst blood vessel. She described this experience in a TED talk entitled "My Stroke of Insight" that has been viewed millions of times (you can watch it yourself at www.ted.com). For example, she perceived herself less and less as a clearly defined being and more as "enormous and expansive and at one with all the energy". She describes this part of her experience as "beautiful" and expresses the wish that her listeners will more often make the conscious choice to take a more "right-brain" perspective that is "at one with all that is".

The brain on auto-pilot

Underneath the cortex there are several areas that are clearly distinct from it, such as the cerebellum, which is located at the back of the head. One of the functions of the cerebellum is to control automatized movement sequences that we hardly need to be consciously aware of. Anybody who can remember what it was like when they first began to learn to drive is familiar with this. In the first few lessons it seemed to require superhuman capacities to keep your eyes on the traffic and turn the steering wheel while at the same time using the pedals and clutch, and possibly even putting the indicators on. If you haven't driven much since you passed your test, you may still break out in a sweat if you have to sit behind the wheel again. But at some point most of us have got the hang of all these procedures and now we could do them all in our sleep. If you ever feel the desire to remind yourself of what the cerebellum is capable of, go to a country where they drive on the opposite side of the road, and rent a car there!

The part of the brain that is oldest in evolutionary terms is located in front of the cerebellum. It is the brainstem, which connects with the spinal cord. The brainstem determines the basic tonus of the arousal of the brain and thus how alert it is. It also maintains the most fundamental bodily functions – respiration, the heart beat and blood pressure – without which we could not survive. Respiration plays a special role because we can consciously change how we breathe. For example, it has been shown to have a calming effect if we deliberately breathe in deeply and then breathe out again slowly.

2. MESSAGES FROM THE DEEP

THE SUBCONSCIOUS

Right in the center of the brain lies a structure which is also very old in evolutionary terms: the limbic system. It consists of many modules and ventricles. While each of them fulfills a specific task, they all work closely together. It is usually this region that is meant when we speak of "the subconscious". It is the center of the autonomic nervous system and thus regulates all our basic bodily functions which don't need any conscious intervention, including body temperature, the need for sleep, digestion, appetite and feeling satiated. This is the source of our instincts and drives, fears and desires – in other words the roots of all feelings, however complex they may be. Because it is precisely this unconscious part of our brain functions that is influenced by neurofeedback it is worth taking a closer look at it.

> The autonomic nervous system consists of a stimulating part and a relaxing part. The "gas pedal" is called the sympathetic nervous system and the "brake" the parasympathetic nervous system. When people are suffering from stress the system gets out of true because the sympathetic nervous system is overly stimulated.

Feelings are embodied thoughts

Most people make a clear distinction between thinking and feeling. Thoughts are "in the head" – for some people they develop mainly in the form of an inner voice and for others more as images; it is rare for other sensory impressions to be predominant. In contrast, feelings have a different quality. The stronger they are, the more they are expressed in the whole of our bodies. Our stomachs become knotted, our voices tremble, our legs turn to jelly. If we look more closely at how these effects arise we will suddenly become aware that thoughts and feelings are closely connected and constantly influence each other in a lively exchange between the mind and the body.

There's no such thing as a rational decision

Sometimes our feelings really seem to get in the way! Imagine, for example, that you are offered a new job which is better paid, but you will have to move to a different department. You'll be expected to take on exciting new tasks, but there will also be other tasks that aren't so much in your line. Should you risk it? You make lists of the pros and cons but that doesn't really help. You do want a change but when you imagine it, it somehow doesn't feel quite right. If only you could simply come to a decision in a matter-of-fact way, without your feelings constantly getting in the way!

But the truth is that it's impossible to make a purely rational decision. We can see this in the example of a man who had to have brain tissue removed from the frontal region of his brain and was subsequently unable to perceive his feelings. Both Elliott's (this is the name the patient is called by in the medical literature) intellectual capacities and his memory remained intact after the operation, but he was no longer able to lead a normal life. Because the connection between his limbic system and frontal cortex had been cut he could no longer weigh up or evaluate anything. Suddenly he was overwhelmed by such a simple question as whether he wanted a cup of coffee or a cup of tea. Although he was still able to work out solutions for problems and develop arguments for and against different alternatives, none of them felt "righter" to him than the others. He also no longer had any wishes or goals, and no rumbling in his gut warning him not to trust a hollow promise or be taken in by a swindler.

So it is probably the lesser of two evils to have to struggle with contradictory feelings from time to time – and perhaps also sometimes to make a decision that in retrospect doesn't seem so wise.

Imagine you walk round a corner and suddenly see a dog. The sensory impression is first transmitted to your thalamus, which is a "distributer" in the limbic system that retransmits the image along two different routes: to the cortex and to the amygdala, the fear center. What the cortex receives is initially a neutral piece of information (something like "animal, large, 6 feet away"), and then this is compared with our inner archive: what kind of animal, what's its body language telling me, do I know it or not. This process takes time – too long if it's a dog that's known to be aggressive and that sees you as an intruder.

Every stimulus is therefore subjected to a rapid check in the amygdala and immediately assigned a very simple emotion that one might translate as "like" or "don't like", the intensity of which may lie anywhere between the extremes of excitement and desire, and panic and disgust. The amygdala knows very well what to think of the dog's bared teeth! The danger signal again takes two routes. It is transmitted to the cortex for conscious perception, while at the same time triggering the appropriate reactions in the body through the secretion of noradrenaline and other stress hormones in preparation for fight or flight. Involuntarily you start. What you are aware of is that your heart starts to beat wildly or you begin to breathe faster.

In the meantime your cortex has sized up the situation and has come to the conclusion that this is Merlin, your neighbor's friendly Australian shepherd dog who has a special ability to "grin". So although his teeth are bared it's not a threat, but an amicable welcome. Danger over! This realization is also assigned an emotion, and this time it's a very positive one. The neurotransmitters that are released produce a powerful feeling of well-being. More complex feelings can then develop if you continue to switch back and forth between the thought and emotion centers. For example, you may feel guilty ("I keep forgetting to give the Smiths back their hedge cutters"), sad ("I would so like to have a dog, too") or happy ("That's great that Merlin is better now!").

From this example we can see that our mind assesses what the encounter with the dog means – and by no means all of its appraisals have to do with the actual situation. This becomes even clearer if the brain first has to figure out a meaning. The release of a small amount of adrenaline initially produces an unspecific arousal which we experience as a slight tingling in the belly – but is that fearful expectation or joyful anticipation? Research has shown that that can be purely a matter of interpretation. In one study men were induced under a pretext to cross a rickety swing bridge in order to get to an attractive female assistant. A much larger number of these participants developed erotic feelings for the woman than did those who had to do with her without having experienced an adrenaline thrill. Similar results were obtained in some other studies in which people who did not know each other had to solve problems together in pairs.

Many more of the subjects fell in love with each other when even only a little excitement and danger was involved.

Stimuli from inside the body, e.g. a fall in blood sugar, can also trigger feelings. These feelings are also registered in the limbic system, they trigger desires (in this case for food), make people restless and motivate them to do something. Pleasant feelings are produced simply by performing an action, and when the original need is finally met there is a feeling of satisfaction. The problem is that the impulses of the body are often not registered in consciousness in the form of a clear statement, but rather as a kind of whining. We may feel that we are not in the best of moods – but what is it in fact that we need? Nutrients, fresh air, exercise, sleep, human contact? Many people are in fact so preoccupied with cognitive problem-solving and so little accustomed to listening to their bodies that they have lost all natural awareness of their own needs.

Another source of feelings are thoughts. You are probably familiar with the situation where you are enjoying sitting in the sun and everything is in fact relaxed but inwardly, you are in a complete turmoil because your boss has ordered you to come in for an "urgent talk". But what is less well-known is how strongly the brain's propensity to produce dark or light thoughts at any one time is dependent on posture, facial expression and gestures. We owe this insight to a relatively young field of psychological research which is currently investigating, under the heading of "embodiment," how the body and the psyche affect each other reciprocally. Smartphones provide us with a good example of what that means in practical terms. If you use your phone to send texts or to access the internet or play games, your head is usually bowed over. This is a posture that is typical when we have negative feelings such as sadness, anxiety and feelings of guilt. Many people also narrow their eyes to help them see the characters on the screen better. In so doing they activate their facial muscles, which contract, as when we are angry or worried about something.

Such information about the state of the body – where it is positioned in a space and which muscles are strongly contracted – is registered by the subconscious on an ongoing basis. This feedback is also known as body feedback and prepares us for mental perception and action. If you sit with your shoulders slumped and simultaneously wrinkle your forehead you are sending a signal to your brain that it must be ready to cope with negative environmental conditions. You will then be more likely to remember a fight than a reconciliation and to be annoyed if it rains instead of being glad that you thought to bring your umbrella. So it's less the objective circumstances that send your mood spiraling downwards than the fact that you are narrowing your perception through your facial expression and body posture. In the same way, adopting a bent-over posture can make your self-confidence crumble and make a task seem more difficult than it might otherwise appear. But it can also work the other way round. The world looks much brighter if we smile – even if at first our smile is totally inauthentic and only produced by holding a pencil between our teeth. And if we assume an inviting posture with rounded arms (as if holding an enormous ball) we become more receptive to inspiration and creative ideas.

3. THE NERVOUS SYSTEM

BEING FULLY CONNECTED

After this brief tour of the most important "sights" of the brain you will want to know how the brain produces all these functions. In order to get an idea of how that works we need to take a closer look at the cells.

Constantly electrified

The brain is densely packed with 100 thousand million nerve cells (neurons), no less than three quarters of which are packed into in the neocortex. Although there are different kinds of neurons, they all have the same basic structure: they consist of a cell body or soma with more than a thousand branches (dendrites), via which both excitatory and inhibiting impulses are received. Each cell also possesses a long extension by means of which impulses can be transmitted to other cells. These extensions are called axons. They can have branches and enter into contact with up to 10,000 other cells. Thus even a single nerve cell has so many different ways of combining that it can be involved in several million information pathways.

The structure of nerve cells and synapses

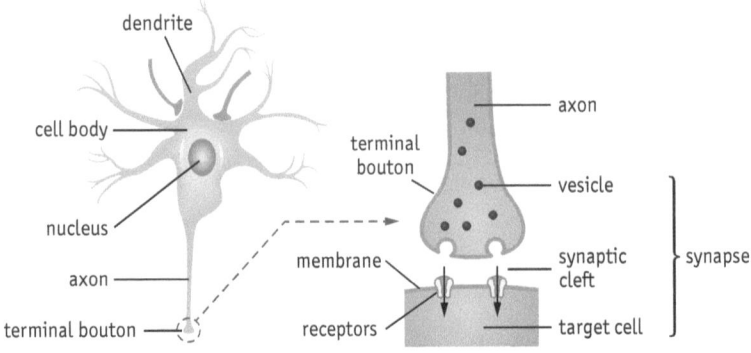

The nerve cells receive signals from other nerve cells via the dendrites and retransmit them via the axons. The terminal bouton stores neurotransmitters in small bubbles or vesicles. When a signal arrives, the vesicles fuse with the membrane of the axon and empty their content into the synaptic cleft. The neurotransmitters can then bind to receptors in the membrane of the target cell, thus triggering a new electrical impulse, and transmit the signal onwards in this way.

If you are imagining the signals as electric wires or telephone cables you're not far off. The signals are in fact transmitted electrically across long distances. This is possible because the membrane of a cell isolates its interior from the fluid surrounding it. The electric potentials inside and outside of the membrane arise from the concentrations of charged molecules (ions). The most important roles are played by the minerals sodium, chloride, potassium and calcium, which can only flow in and out of the cell through special channels in the membrane.

When a neuron is in the resting state its interior is slightly negatively charged. However, the signals that arrive in the cell can change that: they stimulate the ion channels to open and release more positively charged molecules into the cell. In contrast, inhibitory signals strengthen the negative charges. Only when the excitatory signals are clearly in the majority and the positive charge exceeds a certain threshold value is what is known as the action potential generated. This is a new electrical impulse that races down the axon, its strength remaining constant, and finally reaches the cells connected with it. In this way an ingenious system ensures that the information can only move in one direction. The nerve cell subsequently restores its original resting potential in order to be ready for the next activation as quickly as possible.

Voltages are generated by charged molecules

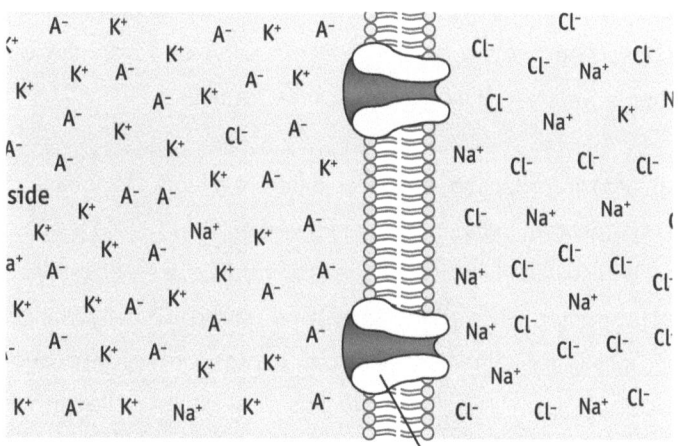

As a result of the distribution of the potassium (K^+), sodium (Na^+) and chloride (Cl^-) ions and other negatively charged molecules (anions, A^-) there is a slightly negative charge between the interior of the cell and the fluid surrounding it. The condition of the pores in the cell membrane determines to what extent to which ions are exchanged.

Neurotransmitters cross the synaptic cleft

However, only in exceptional cases can the electrical impulse simply jump across to the next cell at the end of the "cable". As a rule it first has to be transformed into a chemical signal. This is because there is a cleft between the broadened end of the axon (the terminal bouton) and the target cell. This cleft, together with the structures provided by the two cells, is called the synapse. Neurotransmitters contained in the terminal boutons of the axon are triggered by the incoming impulses and released into the cleft. They cross the intermediate space and bind to the appropriate receptors on the surface of the target cell. You can best imagine these receptors as locks and the neurotransmitters as the keys that unlock them. In this image the doors are the ion channels. When they are opened the charge of the target cell changes – and, just as described above, again a new electrical impulse only arises when the sum of all incoming signals provides sufficient stimulation. Thus the system combines two different principles: it benefits simultaneously from the speed of the electrical transmission and from the built-in "stoppers" with which the signals can be regulated.

The neurotransmitters have various different effects. Dopamine plays an important role in the control of movements. If too little is secreted, as is the case in Parkinson's Disease, for instance, the person will have a strong tremor, while at the same time having difficulty in initiating a purposeful movement. Their facial expression will also become increasingly rigid. Dopamine also has an excitatory effect on many areas of the brain and it controls conscious attention. This neurotransmitter also plays an important role as part of the reward system. The brain secretes more of it when a goal is attained – and that creates feelings of well-being.

There is also much discussion about serotonin, its being described as a "well-being hormone". It has a pleasant stimulating effect and harmonizes the neuronal networks. As a result it creates a feeling of vitality and a positive mood. Serotonin is produced from the protein component tryptophan, which is relatively rare and also has to compete with the other amino-acids for transport across the blood-brain barrier. It can cross it more easily if the metabolism has just been provided with a large amount of sugar or fat – no wonder we don't reach for carrots but for chocolate cookies when we feel in need of comfort.

Enkephalins and endorphins also contribute to our feeling of well-being. They reduce pain and can induce a deep feeling of calm. In contrast, noradrenaline (or norepinephrine) stimulates an inner tingling sensation and makes us alert and attentive to everything that is happening. This can be experienced as a pleasant feeling of anticipation, but also as an uneasy feeling – and, when it is intensified, either as a stimulating "high" or as panic. Startle reactions – as when something makes us jump or we have the feeling that our heart is in our mouth – are mediated in particular by noradrenaline. And finally, you are probably familiar with the neurotransmitter glutamate mainly in its role as a flavor enhancer. It is in fact the most important stimulating neurotransmitter and the one that is most widely distributed across the brain. For example, it supports the connections between neurons and enables us to learn. However, it would be a mistake to believe that we would be able to learn the Italian vocabulary we need for our vacation faster if we ate more foods spiced up with the additive glutamate. In excess, glutamate can even have a lethal effect on nerve cells! However, there is much controversy as to whether glutamate consumed in food also presents such a risk.

The brain's biorhythm

An addition to the neurons themselves a quite different type of cell, the glial cells or glia, are also involved in the regulation of electrical signals. It used to be thought that they were not much more than a kind of insulating and supporting tissue, but in fact they are partners of the nerve cells and of equal value. In the vicinity of the synapses they can even release neurotransmitters themselves, thus enhancing or attenuating signals. They also regulate the energy balance of the brain.

Both of these mechanisms have an influence on how excitable the brain is at any one time. You know what it is like sometimes when you are fully awake and easily able to grasp complex relationships, switch rapidly from one subject to another and get every point immediately. And then a little later your thoughts seem so sticky and dense that even such a simple thing as agreeing on a date to meet becomes a challenge. That's not crazy, but just the normal effects of your biorhythm. The human brain is not a computer that always functions in exactly the same way. It has to regenerate itself from time to time. Evidently the activity of the glia determines both the sleep-wake cycle and the ups and downs of our mental capacities over the course of the day. Typically we will experience a low roughly every 90 to 120 minutes and will need a break. The different sleep phases also change about every 90 minutes.

The human brain is not constantly "online" but needs to "go on standby" from time to time. This is decisive for healthy brain function. We will keep returning to this fact later on in the book.

4. NETWORKS

BRAIN FUNCTIONS ARE TEAMWORK

Millions of electrical impulses shoot through our brains and our bodies every second. They produce the perception of "green" when we look at leaves and one of pain when the soup in our mouths is too hot. They bring about the release of digestive enzymes and make us raise our eyebrows when we are surprised. They conjure up memories of our first kiss and the image of our future dream house, etc. etc. For every impression, every inner impulse and every twitch of a muscle, countless nerve cells have to be activated together in specific patterns. In terms of complexity this is similar to that of an intricate piece of music that only unfolds when all the various instruments are played together in a coordinated way.

Learning and memory

Neurons also fire in defined patterns when thoughts arise. For instance, if you become conscious of the word "kick", the region of the cortex that is responsible for movement reacts. If football has personal meaning for you, the word can even produce a whole flood of other associations. But where are these memories stored in your brain?

In fact there are several "archives". For example, semantic memory collects factual knowledge, e.g. the fact that the Leaning Tower is in Pisa, whereas your memory of the time you visited this town in Tuscany is stored in autobiographic (episodic) memory: it was hot and after viewing that world-famous building you almost left your camera behind in a café. These two archives are also called "declarative" because we are quite familiar with their contents and can describe them. In contrast, procedural memory produces sequences of movement that we no longer have to think about, from walking upright to brushing our teeth. Anxieties and cravings also affect us on an unconscious level. When you actually only intended to fill up at the gas station, but have a bag of croissants in your hand when you get back into the car after paying, your appetite has been stimulated by the smell and look of the croissants – by the memory of how good they taste with butter and honey.

Although recollections are probably not stored in the brain like geological layers, every memory needs to have a special structure in the brain, so that it can create patterns of recollections and reactivate them again later. Science owes this insight in particular to the case of a man who lost his ability to store new information in his brain after undergoing an operation that had serious consequences (see box).

Forever 27

On September 1, 1953 the clock stopped for Henry Molaison, a 27-year-old American who suffered from epilepsy. One day in late summer he decided to undergo brain surgery in the hope that it would control his epilepsy, which was severe. A piece of the temporal lobe was removed on each side of his brain. While he did subsequently have fewer seizures, he paid a very high price: as a result of the operation, at the age of 27, he lost his ability to form new memories. Whatever he did was completely erased from his consciousness after only a few minutes, although he was still able to remember his past – up to 1953. For the whole time during which he collaborated with scientists this was always his answer when asked what the current year was. There came a point when on looking at himself in the mirror he would see an old man looking back at him with whom he was hardly able to identify, because he still believed he was only twenty-seven. He would understand his doctors' explanation – only to forget it shortly afterwards.

Today we know that it is the hippocampus, which is located inside the temporal lobe and part of the limbic system, that forms lasting memories from the fleeting impressions of the short-term memory. Henry Molaison's case also provided brain researchers with some other insights, one of which being the existence of procedural memory. This was discovered when they observed that Molaison was able to master motor skill tasks better each time he performed them, even though he couldn't remember having practiced them. He was also able to remember some facts from the time before his operation, but not a single personal memory. On the day he died in December 2008 he still thought it was 1953 and he was 27 years old.

Most memories are not virtual reality versions of the original situation, but are modified every time they are reactivated. This is a bit like what happens when we play the game "Chinese whispers" or "Telephone". Most of us find it hard to accept that our memories are not infallible, but the research results on this are clear. And yet there seems to be more to this than meets the eye, since when individual brain areas are over-stimulated – whether by targeted electric stimulation during surgery or by epileptic discharges – sometimes extremely detailed, isolated memories arise. They are crystal clear and seem as real as holographic projections. Perhaps many – or all? – memories are stored in such detail and it's just that under normal circumstances they are not recalled in their entirety.

However, it is probably the case that most impressions are not committed to memory at all. The nerve cells fire but the activation pattern soon disappears – as if somebody was using water to draw on hot asphalt. Memories only form if the patterns can be linked to something that is already known or if they are often repeated. These processes also take place during sleep and encode the events of the day. Impressions that have been received under favorable circumstances are particularly easily memorized. In most cases this means that a lot of feeling was involved, even if it was only the thrill of the encounter with something new.

This also explains why many people become less and less open to new things, the older they get. The more a person has already experienced, the more their brain tends to make life easy for itself and rely on its store of previous experiences. If allowed to, it will always try to find energy-saving routines. If we want to lure it outside of its comfort zone into new territory we must offer it something that feels better to it – like enthusiasm, for example. If you decide to go through your day with your eyes wide open, looking for things that are joyful or make you curious and bolster your enthusiasm, you will find such things – and create wonderful new memories much more often.

Neurofeedback also gives the brain an impulse that helps it to leave the beaten track and try out new reaction patterns.

On the level of neuronal activity patterns it makes no difference to the brain whether it carries out actions itself, whether it remembers them or whether it sees others performing them, and so without consciousness we would have no chance of being able to distinguish our fantasies from the world outside our heads. Scientists find it difficult to define consciousness because all attempts to explain it at least touch on spiritual modes of thinking. However, it seems certain that three networks play a decisive role in the development of consciousness.

Brief downtimes and alert attention

Three of the networks known to brain research today are of particular interest for neurofeedback. The technical term for one of these is the "default mode network", which is a resting-state network. The default mode always becomes active when nothing is happening that captures the interest of the brain. Our attention then turns inward and the brain occupies itself (with itself) and allows the mind to wander. This will be familiar to you because this state is completely normal, it occurs countless times a day, e.g. in the doctor's waiting room, when you're brushing your teeth or when a parents' association meeting drags on for ever. However, the ability to disconnect from the outside world and not really be mentally present at all isn't particularly well regarded. It's all too easy to be seen as addle-brained, dozy or even a bit dim-witted – especially since mindfulness is en vogue right now, even when you're washing the breakfast dishes.

It is certainly a good idea for us to give our full attention to a task and be truly present in the here-and-now, but it is equally important to allow ourselves to pay attention to thoughts that wander aimlessly, to wild ideas and incoherent snippets of memory. The default mode network has to become active in order for us to process impressions and experiences and to develop a subjective attitude towards them. We need this in order to be able to learn from our experiences and shape our future – and so that we don't just keep repeating old habits, but also sometimes develop creative new ways.

Meditation activates the default mode network

Many people struggle with the fact that they do not grow calm when they turn their attention inward during meditation and that on the contrary, the noise in their heads gets especially loud when they do this. This is also the activity of the resting state network. It is perceived as unpleasant in this situation because it becomes clear to us that many of our thoughts are only useless chatter and often also rather negative. However, if we were to fight against them it would be like trying to smooth the surface of an expanse of water by banging on the waves. And it is also not the goal of meditation to achieve complete quiet, particularly not for beginners. Rather, the idea is not to be completely at the mercy of our inner turbulence. When we meditate we practice simply allowing our thoughts to pass by, thus achieving an inner peace.

We could also see the default setting as a kind of immune system of the psyche, since these states provide the brain with brief periods of respite that allow it to create order and organize itself — like a mini-version of the extensive clean-up tasks that have to take place when we are asleep. This is probably why the brain lowers its level of arousal every 90 to 120 minutes during the day, affording itself a little slack. And maybe that's why it feels so good to stare into a camp fire, gaze up at a starry sky or sit by a babbling brook. But most people experience such moments far too rarely. Nowadays all these little downtimes for the mind are increasingly disappearing, because every time there's even the tiniest gap in our daily routine we immediately reach for our phones.

But of course when the brain is functioning healthily it creates a balance between looking dreamily inward and the ability to react to the outside world in an alert and concentrated way. Our central attention network (referred to in the technical terminology as the "central executive network", CEN) plays a major role in this. Ideally, a person can switch rapidly between the two states – inward- or outward-focused – adapting to the situation as required. When you're staring into space in the doctor's waiting room while in your mind you're wandering along a beach on a Pacific island, you will of course want to be able to switch over immediately and be aware of your surroundings when the receptionist calls you. This abrupt switch is made possible by the salience network (SN), which monitors the situation and decides whether a stimulus is important enough for you to turn your attention outward. You can completely tune out the piped music that's coming out of the speakers in the waiting room, and with a bit of luck even the grousing of a child with a cold won't distract you from your vacation fantasy. But as soon as your name is called, you'll be back from the island in an instant and ready to talk through your lab results with your doctor. So the salience network acts as a filter.

> In order to be able to switch quickly between day-dreaming and focused attention we need to be rested. The more exhausted we are, the stronger the stimuli from outside need to be to get through to us.

In recent years there have been increasing indications that many mental disturbances arise because these networks are not working well together. Thus, for example, in people with autism the attention network is also activated when the brain should actually be relaxed and also somewhat cut off from the external world. But it makes life very exhausting if we are constantly at the mercy of a flood of stimuli.

It also makes it impossible to switch from a narrow, concentrated focus to a relaxed, expansive mode of perception in which we are able to recognize connections and find creative solutions. In contrast, people with depression seem rather to be too withdrawn into themselves.

Research on neurofeedback indicates that this is precisely where the more modern forms of this kind of therapy intervene. They train the brain to better control its own excitability and switch more easily from one state to the other – just as each individual situation requires. The next section of this book describes the different versions of this training.

PART 2

NEUROFEEDBACK – A MACHINE WORKOUT FOR THE BRAIN

When neurofeedback is mentioned, three fundamentally different approaches that need to be clearly distinguished from one another are often lumped together. In this section you will discover more about the three types of training and how they differ from each other. The most important thing they have in common is that to clients they all seem easy and fun.
In Part 3 of the book you will then find details of the main problems and disorders that can be treated effectively.

The previous chapters gave you a brief overview of the organization of the brain and how the individual nerve cells transmit their information. The electrical activity generated can be measured by attaching sensors (electrodes) to the scalp and connecting them to a receiver. Individual nerve impulses are not recorded, as the signals they emit are too weak. However that isn't necessary, since, as you know, notable effects only arise when thousands of nerve cells fire simultaneously. The recording is called the EEG (electroencephalograph) and it shows characteristic wave patterns, called frequencies. The diagram "Waves and frequencies" shows what is meant by this.

Waves and frequencies

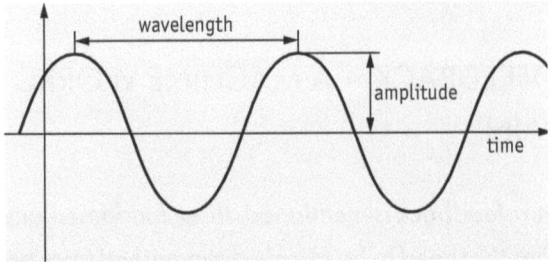

On the physical level two parameters are mainly used to describe waves. The heights of the peaks of the waves (amplitude) show the strength of the individual impulses, and the wavelengths (the distance between one peak and the next) determine the length of time between two peaks. Frequency is measured by the number of waves per second (Hertz or Hz).

So how does neurofeedback work? The principle is always the same, as is shown in the next diagram – the electrodes measure selected brain currents and transmit them to a computer. The computer then integrates the information into a film, which the client is asked to watch on the screen. The animations, images and scenes will change depending on brain activity. This is the feedback which reflects back to the brain what it is doing in the moment. The feedback varies in accordance with the three forms of neurofeedback. While it may be clearly recognizable and is sometimes even reinforced by additional features such as a smiley as a reward, it can also be so subtle that the patient is mainly aware of it on the subconscious level. You can find out more about this in later chapters.

The wired-up client

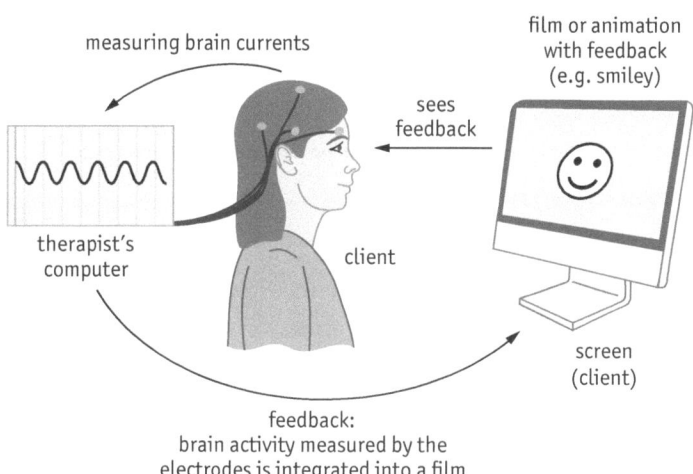

measuring brain currents

film or animation with feedback (e.g. smiley)

sees feedback

therapist's computer

client

screen (client)

feedback:
brain activity measured by the
electrodes is integrated into a film

In neurofeedback the principle is always the same – the client watches a film or an animation on their screen. What they see is changed by the computer in accordance with the brain signals that are measured.

The feedback is like a mirror for the brain in which it can recognize its own activity and then try out how changes affect it. This works because the subconscious is able to perceive a vast number of impressions at any one time and to very quickly discover patterns and regularities. It therefore has no difficulty in recognizing the changes in its own state mirrored in what is happening on the screen. It uses this external information to regulate its own activity in exactly the same way as it uses internal signals. You will have experienced this if you have tried to balance on one leg. The more abnormal you find a position, the less you can rely merely on an internal feeling about where you are in the room – you are dependent on additional information conveyed by your eyes. Try holding the "tree" position in yoga – it's much easier to keep your balance when your eyes are open and your brain can orient itself towards fixed objects in your field of vision in order to keep correcting your posture.

But even then you need practice. Whether their eyes are open or not, in their first yoga sessions hardly anyone stands elegant and upright like a beech tree when doing "the tree", most look much more like a mountain pine waving in the wind. It is the same with neurofeedback – even with external feedback the brain first has to learn and train how to best achieve a desired result.

> The possibility to control a computer with the aid of brain activity is also used to support people with total paralysis. With a BCI (Brain Computer Interface) they can learn to use a cursor to select letters or words on a screen and thus to communicate with others and to operate equipment.

How the brain actually manages to do this remains just as inaccessible to the conscious mind as how we manage to keep our balance while standing on one leg and reaching our arms above our heads at the same time.

What is biofeedback?

Biofeedback used to be used as an umbrella term for all different forms of feedback training. Today it is has become accepted that biofeedback should only be used to refer to those forms of therapy in which bodily reactions are visualized by means of a computer – and not, as in neurofeedback, the activity of the brain. The most frequently used parameters are muscle tension, pulse, skin temperature and skin conductance (this shows if someone is nervous and that is why they are sweating). For example, a common cause of tension head-aches is tense neck muscles. The feedback system can show patients when they involuntarily tense their muscles and when they have found a way to totally release them. In time, these new reactions become just as much an unconscious habit as the old unhealthy ones were.

Many people find the idea of being wired up and influenced by a computer quite unsettling. But it is not that you are "reprogrammed" or data is being "stored" in your brain. Children, especially, feel almost disappointed by this because they quite often hope that after the treatment they will be good at math without having to make an effort. However, the training doesn't mean that you don't have to learn, but "only" that it will be easier to learn or even possible to learn at all.

Unlike electric or magnetic field therapies, neurofeedback does not require the brain to be exposed to any currents or fields.

Likewise, a person's personality is not fundamentally altered by the therapy. If you are impulsive you will still tend to be so – but you won't be completely at the mercy of your impulsiveness. What the training will do is enable you to decide whether you want to act on the impulse or not. Some people describe the change in themselves as a return to who they really are and say things like "Now I'm much more myself again". But before we start considering what can be achieved by neurofeedback in concrete terms, in the next three chapters we will begin by describing the three different forms of the training.

1. CONFIDENTLY RIDING THE WAVES

FREQUENCY BAND TRAINING

The brain waves shown in the EEG are divided into six groups, or frequency bands. These are usually referred to by the Greek letters: alpha, beta, delta, theta and gamma. In addition there is also a frequency band that is abbreviated to SMR, which is linked to the story of its discovery (see Part 3). Several frequencies always appear in an EEG, but it is possible to see from the specific combination and also the height of the peaks of the waves what state the brain is in at a particular moment – i.e. whether it is focused or drowsy, alarmed or relaxed. The EEG also gives clear indications as to what arousal state the brain is in at any one moment – the scientific term for this is "vigilance".

> It is still often assumed that the frequencies in the EEG give an absolutely truthful picture of a person's state, but it's not that simple. It can even be the case that what any one of the frequency bands patterns shows deviates substantially from the state a person is currently in. For this reason the readings must always be viewed in conjunction with the patient's subjective experience of their current state.

The different brain waves

The slow waves of the theta frequency band (4 – 7 Hz, see following table) are characteristic of deep relaxation or drowsiness. In deep sleep the delta waves dominate, and these are even slower (1-3 Hz). Many theta band frequencies also occur in meditative states. If one needs to concentrate on a task, however, it is not desirable to have a large proportion of theta waves.

When the brain is relaxed and awake, but not focusing on anything in particular, the EEG shows the alpha waves as being dominant, in the range of 8 – 12 Hz. It is predominantly in the borderline range between the theta and alpha states that the mind is very open to information from the subconscious and receptive to ideas and new ways of solving problems.

The SMR frequencies (12 – 15 Hz) are particularly interesting. They appear on the EEG more frequently when the brain is relaxed but also focused and ready for action. Clients particularly like to achieve this state because their performance is then at its best, regardless of whether it is a question of scoring at football, memorizing vocabulary, following a lecture or playing a challenging piece on the violin.

The more someone applies themselves to a task in a focused and deliberate way, the more one finds the faster beta frequency waves of 15-20 Hz in the EEG. If the still faster waves of 20 – 30 Hz appear, this is often a sign of extreme tension, which tends to constrict thinking more and more – this is typical of anxiety and other stress states. However, at over 30 Hz, in the gamma wave range, something quite new happens. These frequencies often occur in states of consciousness that practiced meditators experience, for example. They experience the mind as quite still and clear – as if detached from the body. However, these impressions can also occur in states of panic, in which case they are often experienced in a very negative way.

The categories of brain wave frequencies

Name	Frequencies	State of arousal
Delta	1 – 3 Hz	deep sleep
Theta	4 – 7 Hz	drowsy, trance-like
Alpha	8 – 12 Hz	awake, dreamy, inattentive
SMR	12 – 15 Hz	relaxed, but focused and attentive
(Low) Beta	15 – 20 Hz	very focused, alert
High Beta	20 – 30 Hz	tense, high stress level
Gamma	over 30 Hz	In a state of contemplation, but clear, as though "disembodied"

Watching TV can be therapeutic

The first neurofeedback applications used the discoveries described above to develop what is called SMR-Beta Training, in which users practice keeping themselves in a relaxed but alert state. Each session lasts 20 – 30 minutes. On the technical level they receive feedback on how the mixture of brain waves is developing in their brain. The goal is to achieve three changes: firstly a reduction in the proportion of those frequencies that are connected with mind-wandering or zoning out (theta) and restlessness (high beta), secondly an increase in the proportions of SMR and low beta frequencies, and thirdly an increase in the amplitude (the peaks of the waves).

In the early years of neurofeedback, clients would receive the feedback only in the form of simple sounds and bar charts. In addition, a sun or smiley would pop us if the desired thresholds were exceeded.

Nowadays there are more sophisticated ways of providing the feedback. The client can watch an entertaining film or an episode of their favorite TV series – however, this pleasant entertainment only runs without interruption for as long as the brain remains in a relaxed, alert mode. As soon as it tries hard to concentrate or the mind wanders, the images start to falter. This can be really frustrating, and of course the brain waves associated with frustration have an even stronger braking effect. The video only continues when the brain returns to wakeful calm, and soon the client has learned to keep the film running smoothly. This is clearly a more effective reward for the brain than seeing a smiley for the nth time.

Although SMR-Beta Training is still used today, mainly in the treatment of concentration problems, it has actually become outdated. In many therapy practices it is now merely a "treat" at the end of the real training to keep children on board – most of them think it's cool if watching a bit of TV counts as therapy.

On the other hand there are still good reasons to use other forms of frequency band training. In alpha synchrony training clients practice keeping large sections of the brain in synchrony in a calm alpha rhythm. The more successful this is, the deeper the relaxation. This form of training is good particularly for people who find it hard to "wind down". With gamma synchrony training it is possible to go even deeper into meditative states.

In contrast, the goal of Alpha/Theta training (A/T training), is to practice staying in between these frequency bands and thus attain a trance-like state. This is not only immensely relaxing and restorative, but also the gateway to deeper sleep stages. Some people have disturbed sleep because they are unable to simply let go and enter this state. The moment they reach it, unpleasant images and sensations rise up out of the unconscious and they wake with a start. This training can help them to face this problem and process what is bothering them in a safe environment. Moreover, the trance state is particularly suitable for changing inner images and in this way to get a grip on persistent habits, for example.

2. TRAINING THE WATCHDOG

SCP TRAINING

In addition to the frequency bands there are other electrical signals that can be measured by EEG, although, at 0.1 Hz, the waves are much slower. For this reason they have been labeled Slow Cortical Potentials, or SCPs for short. They do not reflect so much the current arousal level of the brain but rather an aspect of excitability, i.e. the readiness to react to a stimulus.

We can understand what this means if we take traffic lights at road-works as an example. Imagine you are sitting in your car at the front of the queue, looking expectantly at the red light, but nothing happens for quite a while. Unless you've just switched on an interesting radio program or some great music your thoughts will probably start to wander – and your readiness potential will sink, and also your response speed. When the light finally does turn amber, your brain will ramp up its excitability (ideally really fast). It has now brought its full attention back to the traffic situation and is preparing itself to become active. Then, as soon as the stimulus "green" appears, you can drive off immediately.

The results of the research to date indicate that the SCPs reflect the activities of the neuronal networks that were introduced in the last section: the resting state network, the central attention or central executive network (CEN) and the salience network (SN). You will remember that the resting state network takes over when awareness is focused inward, i.e. on thoughts, memories and dreams, whereas the CEN is activated when external stimuli require attention. The SN mediates between these states. In SCP training the patient practices raising and lowering the excitability of their brain and being able to reach the level that they need at that particular moment.

Comic figures as training partners

The best way to see what the training is like in practice is to look at a concrete example. Let's assume that our client is Melanie, a nine-year-old girl who has concentration difficulties. Melanie cuddles up under a blanket in a comfortable armchair and has four electrodes attached to her head with a conductive white paste. Today she has chosen Lucky Luke to be her partner in her brain training; it could just as easily have been a different comic figure, or an airplane or a floating balloon or any number of other things.

SCP-Training

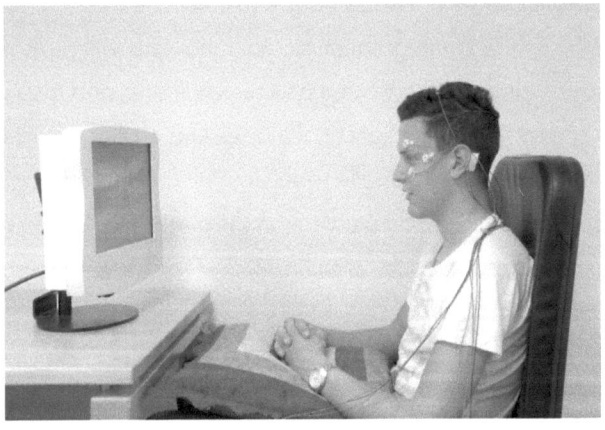

As long as clients have been wired up correctly
they can just sit back and relax.

In a scene lasting eight seconds Lucky Luke rides from left to right, and this sequence is repeated 80 to 120 times during a therapy session. Before each trial, an arrow appears in the middle of the screen, pointing either upwards or downwards. This arrow shows Melanie what she has to do for the next eight seconds, i.e. use the strength of her brain signals to move the figure on the screen either up or down. And then Lucky does not simply ride to the right, but, as instructed, he goes uphill at the same time. Done it! This achievement alone is very satisfying for the brain, but there is an additional reward as well – in the middle of the screen the grinning face of Lucky's dog pops up. In other clips it might be a smiley or a sun. And then a new trial begins, regardless of whether the target was met or not.

Whenever Melanie steers her figure upwards she has also raised her readiness potential, i.e. made her brain ready for action – and vice versa. As a rule steering both up and down are practiced equally frequently; it is only in some conditions such as epilepsy that the weighting can be different.

A training session always includes something that might be called transfer trials. When this happens, although Melanie receives an instruction as to the direction she has to shift her inner state, initially she gets no feedback. It is only at the end of the trial that she will see reflected back to her, by the reward sign popping up (Lucky's grinning dog or a sun), whether she has completed the task or not. By means of these trials what has been learned is transferred more successfully into daily life, where there is also no visible feedback for the activity of the brain. Ultimately it should become quite superfluous – in the same way as when you ride a bike, the time comes when you can keep your balance without Dad's hand supporting you.

Melanie also succeeds in directing her screen figures very consistently – but she doesn't know how she does it. To begin with most clients try to direct what is happening deliberately, but that is exactly what won't work. They can – and must – permit themselves to just let go and allow the unconscious part of their brain to guide them. Only then will they succeed in completing the task set and up-or down-regulate the excitability of their brain. It is a bit like practicing very finely adjusting the flame on a gas cooker and making it bigger or smaller as required.

Transfer cards

Transfer cards can also be used as further support in everyday situations. They serve to remind clients of the states that they have learned in the training and in this way they can help them to cope better with situations that they find difficult. These aids may be, for example, laminated copies of the training screen that clients can put into a school bag or wallet. They can then look at them briefly before a test or a meeting with the boss in order to concentrate better or become calmer. Or they might play a helpful video on their phone or conjure up a favorite fantasy image – there is no limit to the creative possibilities.

3. ENCOURAGING THE REORGANIZATION OF THE BRAIN ILF TRAINING

The third form of neurofeedback was developed from frequency band training by the American couple Susan and Siegfried Othmer, who have continued to improve it over a period of 30 years – and are still not thinking of retiring. Therefore the method is also rightfully called the Othmer method.

The signals used here, which have between 100 mHz and 0.005 mHz, are significantly slower than the SCPs, which is why they are also known as Infra Low Frequencies (ILF). From a technical point of view, the term frequency no longer makes any sense in this infra-low range, since a single oscillation would last several hours. If you compare the activity of the brain with the movement of the sea, the frequencies are like the waves rolling in, whereas the SCPs and, even more so, the ILFs correspond rather to the gradual rise and fall of the tide. In ILF training, therapists monitor how steeply the electrical potential rises. If we stay with the sea image, this means how high and how fast the tide comes in.

The ILFs also reflect the excitability of the brain, but if we compare this method with SCP neurofeedback there are several fundamental differences. Firstly, the positioning of the electrodes in ILF training can be varied, so that different areas of the brain can be targeted. Secondly, the method monitors far smaller sections of the electrical activity – these are selected according to the needs of each individual client and then enlarged, as with a magnifying glass. And thirdly, in addition to the slow potentials the activities of the classical frequency bands are integrated into the feedback. All of these details that have been developed over the years make the method much more effective today.

Unconscious learning while playing computer games

In the various forms of frequency band and SCP training clients are consciously aware of whether the task that has been set is successful or not. In ILF training, however, this is not the case. Clients simply watch TV programs or films which can contain nature scenes or ever-changing patterns with a musical backdrop. If clients want more action they can also allow themselves to be riveted by computer games and shoot across the water on virtual jet skis or take sharp corners in racing cars. Nowadays it is even possible for clients to wear special glasses and completely immerse themselves in virtual surroundings, instead of looking at a screen. This gives the brain an even more intense experience.

While this is happening, the electrodes on the client's head register the brain waves in the areas of the brain selected by the therapist, and the program integrates this information into the film. This feedback influences the films in quite different ways. For instance, the height of the waves in the computer game or the brightness of the film or the intensity of the colors in the pattern can change. The volume or the speed of the scene on the screen may also vary. And in addition to the visual and auditory feedback a client can also receive tactile stimuli if, for example, they are holding a vibrating cuddly toy in their hand.

ILF-Training

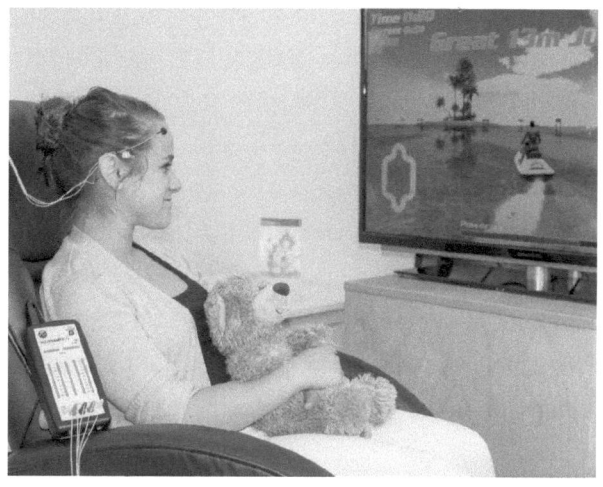

In ILF training clients can either just see and hear their chosen film or also receive tactile (felt) signals from a cuddly toy. If they want to they can also pick up a control device and use it as they would in a computer game. For example, a boat could be steered to the left or right.

Clients often believe they've worked out what the principle behind the feedback is. Then they say something like, "Ah, I get it! When I relax the picture gets brighter!" But firstly they've usually missed the mark and secondly it is actually not necessary to grasp what is happening on a conscious level. The client can just sit back and watch or play a computer game and let their subconscious guide them, because the subconscious is first-rate at discovering patterns and relating them to internal states. The conscious mind can take a break for a while.

It is a totally different scenario for the therapist, however! It is imperative that the therapist is present during the session in order to correct the training settings if the client is experiencing problems. For example, they might start to feel dizzy or sick or really tired. It is not always easy to determine the optimal settings in the individual case – but when they have been found, it simply feels "right" to the client. The mind will usually have difficulty in pinning down this feeling and putting a label on it, but it is nonetheless reliable and can often even be reproduced in subsequent sessions by using the same settings.

This "rightness" can also be evident if the client's mood improves and they become more relaxed and focused. Some people report that they feel really clear and attentive, others say that they experience an inner calm such as they have never experienced before, or at least not for a very long time. Even the liveliest children, and even those who are autistic, often appear quite meditative during the session.

It is also not uncommon for reactions (both positive and negative) to begin to emerge only in the days following a session. It may be that the client sleeps better or their digestion becomes more normal, but it may also be that they have headaches or experience mood swings. For this reason it is preferable for the therapist to be overcautious rather than push too hard and they should always ask clients how they have felt after a session. The changes clients describe are the most important basis for establishing the correct neurofeedback settings. It is like when the optician adjusts the strength of new lenses when we're getting new glasses. She tries out different combinations and takes her lead from the client's feedback when deciding how many diopters they need. What the neurofeedback therapist does is exactly the same.

This is why in ILF training there can be no formal guidelines as to which protocols are best for particular illnesses or symptoms. Different ADHD or migraine patients can be given completely different treatment plans, even when they have similar symptoms! Therapists can in fact draw on shared clinical experience when determining the best places to position the electrodes and assessing which settings will probably be useful.

However, whether these will be appropriate or not in each individual case can only be decided in dialog with their clients or their parents. You will learn more about this approach, known as "symptom tracking", in Part 3 of the book. Another way to ascertain a client's progress is to ask them to do the CPT (Continuous Performance Test, see box).

Continuous Performance Test

This tool can be used to measure how well someone is able to remain focused on something over a long period of time and continue to react appropriately. It involves holding a device in both hands, with both thumbs on a button. In the middle of a small screen, a large square composed of smaller squares appears, the center of which is either empty or full. Depending which of these figures appears, the client's task is either to press one of the buttons or not. As clients do so, the speed with which they recognize the correct figure and the various errors that may occur are measured. If the client keeps pressing the button, even though the wrong image or perhaps no image at all was visible, this is an indication of excessive impulsiveness or impatience. If, on the other hand, they press it very late, this indicates that their attention has strayed.

The test takes 20 minutes, which is a really long time. As time goes on, the images appear increasingly rapidly, only to get slower again towards the end, when the client will have become really bored anyway. Some people find the test so challenging that at the beginning of the neurofeedback training they can hardly keep going till the end.

A big advantage of ILF neurofeedback is that positive changes very quickly become apparent. Whereas other methods usually require 10 – 20 sessions, with ILF training the first effects can often be seen after fewer than five. It must be said that much of the learning takes place "out in the real world". As a result of the changes that they have subconsciously learned to make in their inner state, clients perceive and feel many things differently from the way they did before. The skills they have practiced in training become consolidated when they behave differently in their everyday lives and have positive experiences as a result. This process takes place automatically and in fact requires no further external help. Nevertheless, some clients or their parents still want transfer cards, like the ones used in SCP training. There is no harm in these, but there is no need for them with the ILF method. If the client can only attain the desired state by consciously doing something, the training was not as effective as it could have been.

With ILF neurofeedback, in particular, the therapist's experience and the attention they pay to detail are also very important for the success of the treatment (see box). However, this very fact is a hindrance to the scientific investigation of the method.

How to find a good therapist

For a long time medical training was all that was required to be permitted to buy neurofeedback equipment and then use it to treat patients. That is changing, fortunately, and the equipment for ILF training, at least, and increasingly also for SCP training, can now only be provided to therapists who have learned at least the basic principles of the method in a course lasting several days. The skills of the practitioners are also constantly improving because today there are far more opportunities for further training and supervision.

In ILF training, in particular, the therapist's experience is crucial if the treatment is to be successful. It is also important that he or she takes time, at the beginning in particular, to ask about the client's symptoms and previous history. Another mark of a high quality therapist is that they will not leave a client on their own during the session – the therapist should also be there to intervene if the client starts feeling unwell. The practice of connecting several people to the devices at the same time in different rooms borders on extreme negligence if the result is a kind of "mass production".

Checklist for choosing a therapist
- What neurofeedback method does the therapist use?
- What training have they had?
- Do they consult with other therapists (supervision)?
- How long have they been using the method?
- Do they take a thorough history (ask about symptoms and previous medical history)?
- Do they make unrealistic promises or do they point out that it is never possible to predict how the therapy will progress?
- Do they stay in the room during the treatment?

4. THE STATE OF THE ART IN RESEARCH ON NEUROFEEDBACK

While there are many indications as to what makes the different forms of neurofeedback effective, so far the exact relationships have still not been fully explained. Most of the high quality studies are on SCP training. They have confirmed what research on frequency band training had already shown, i.e. that neurofeedback is mainly effective in the treatment of epilepsy, migraine and ADHD. There is also evidence that the concomitant use of neurofeedback improves the likelihood of a good outcome in addiction therapy. Currently about 150 new scientific studies are published each year, including some very promising ones on tinnitus, sleep problems, tics, autism, brain damage and anxiety disorders.

However, occasionally studies are published that come to the conclusion that that there is no difference between neurofeedback and placebo training. How come? Many scientists simply fail to engage in discussion with the practitioners and do not take into account practical experience in their study designs. Training methods are often still tested in research that many practitioners no longer use – for the very reason that they do not deliver good results.

It is sometimes maintained that there are no studies at all on ILF neurofeedback, but this is in fact not the case. However, the studies often employ methods that have long been outdated.

Another reason is that in studies it is not desirable for there to be a large number of interactions between the therapist and the test person – the researchers want to eliminate all factors that could contaminate the effect of the method itself. They therefore ask the practitioner to talk to the test person as little as possible and in some studies the practitioner even has to leave the room. Yet, in the case of neuro-feedback, removing the therapist in this way has a detrimental effect on the results! And this has nothing to do with any way in which the therapist might influence the test person that could be interpreted as a placebo effect (see box).

The placebo effect: an astonishing achievement of the brain

In studies of the effects of therapies and agents, studies with a double-blind, placebo-controlled design are considered to be the gold standard. In other words, alongside the genuine treatment there is also a "sham" treatment (placebo), and during the trials neither the test persons nor the therapists know who is receiving which treatment. If it is only the test persons who are left in the dark, the design is called "single-blind". The aim of this procedure is to find out which effects result from the therapy, and which are also in part due to the positive expectations of the patients. What in some studies might be considered to be simply a "nuisance" and irrelevant is in fact an interesting phenomenon in itself!

Because today we know that the effects of sham treatments – such as taking pills without any active ingredients – are by no means merely a figment of the imagination. The hope that symptoms will improve produces quantifiable physical reactions, for example the secretion of pain-relieving neurotransmitters or hormones. In its simplest form this is familiar to all of us – a mother kisses the pain away that is caused by a graze on the knee. On a larger scale we can see how powerful this is when a serious illness such as advanced cancer suddenly disappears without any medical explanation.

The reverse is also true – if you don't believe in a therapy its curative effects will be far smaller or non-existent. This is because the brain also reacts to the expectation that something will be useless or possibly even harmful. This is known as the "nocebo effect". Research has shown that even strong medications such as opioids can be completely ineffective if patients do not have a positive attitude towards them. This shows that it is not the therapies that are the decisive factor in someone becoming healthy but the inherent self-organizing capacity that is part of every human being's make up. This capacity enables us to absorb impulses from outside to reorganize ourselves and ideally to feel better as a result. Good therapists, teachers and trainers are well aware of this and take care to fuel this inner strength in their protégés through the way they conduct themselves and communicate.

The placebo effect is thus an important ally in the day-to-day work of a therapist! But it is precisely when a practitioner cannot rely on this that the strengths of neurofeedback become evident. Initially very many clients are very skeptical or even only agree to do the training to prove to a member of their family that the method is just hocus pocus – and yet the method also works in these cases too. This is because the training speaks to the subconscious on a quite elementary level and simply reflects back what the subconscious is doing. Receiving and integrating such impulses is the most ordinary thing in the world for the brain, and unlike with medication and operations, neurofeedback does not compromise its integrity. For this reason it would be quite presumptuous to say that neurofeedback cures anything– what it actually does is put the brain in a position to cure itself.

The ground rule that the more the treatment plan is adapted to the client the better the results, applies particularly to ILF training. Only an experienced therapist who has undergone comprehensive training and proceeds with great care can really exploit the method to the full. With such a complex theory this should not come as a surprise, because we have the same expectations in regard to operations, for example. In the case of surgery, particularly when it comes to complicated procedures, it is also clear that the more skilled and experienced the surgeon is, the better the outcome.

In other words, when you are trying to find the right therapist, the recommendations of other clients who have similar problems to you will be more helpful to you than the findings of research. Many of the fields in which neurofeedback is used have still not been researched systematically, but the therapists have nevertheless already acquired a wealth of experience. In Part 3 you will find out more about the use of ILF neurofeedback in particular for various illnesses and symptoms. Examples of typical real cases are presented to show you what happens during the course of treatment.

More Information

You can find out more about current developments in ILF neurofeedback at www.eeginfo.com/research/index.jsp where you will find an overview of research into the applications and mechanisms of brain self-regulation that underline neurofeedback.

PART 3

HOW NEUROFEEDBACK CAN HELP

ADHD, anxiety disorders, migraine, depression ... How can a single form of treatment be helpful for such different illnesses? In fact, all these disorders have one important thing in common, and that is that the fundamental arousal of the brain and its capacity to regulate itself are not (or no longer) in a healthy balance. And this is exactly where neurofeedback comes in. This part of the book describes in concrete terms what this therapy offers for the treatment of twelve different illnesses and their symptoms. We describe genuine cases from clinical practice to give you an idea of how a client's process can develop.

We have now given you an introduction to the different types of neurofeedback and shown what a complex field this is – and also why to the clients it nonetheless seems like child's play. All they have to do is watch films and animations or play computer games. While they are doing this their brains are learning, unconsciously and quite incidentally, to shift into states that have not previously been so easily accessible. However, the training may still be frustrating to begin with if it takes ten or even twenty sessions to achieve any results.

With ILF neurofeedback it is possible to achieve observable effects much faster than that, often even after only a single session. That is one reason why I work almost exclusively with this method in my practice. I do use frequency band training as well, but only as a complement to ILF neurofeedback. I don't use SCP training at all because it requires different equipment.

SCP training is better for some people because it gives them the feeling that they are actively doing something and staying in control. I refer these clients to trusted colleagues who use SCP training.

This part of the book is almost exclusively about ILF training, because this is the only method that can be adapted to each individual client, and because in my opinion it therefore achieves the best results. But before I go into the details of how the most modern form of neurofeedback treats functional brain disturbances, I would like to remind you of how this form of treatment began. Where did the idea of using electrical brain waves in treatment come from in the first place? After all, originally EEG was used only as a diagnostic tool.

EEGs that can be used for making a diagnosis are much more complex than the comparably simple leads used in neurofeedback.

The history of the therapeutic use of EEG actually began with a number of coincidences, the curiosity of a researcher and the courage of his assistant.

The Birth of Neurofeedback

In the 1960s Barry Sterman, an American psychologist, was doing research in cats on brain waves during different sleep phases. He had trained the cats to lie still and at some point he noticed that when they did so a particular rhythm was visible in the EEG. This rhythm was seen at frequencies of between 12 and 15 Hertz and was similar to the "sleep spindles" that appear during the phase of falling asleep – but the cats were wide awake and alert.

"Sleep spindles" are a brain wave pattern that is detectable in EEGs. They show that the brain is shutting itself off from external stimuli to a great extent in order to be able to stabilize sleep and reach deeper stages.

Sterman called this frequency pattern "SMR", which stands for "sensorimotor rhythm", after the sensorimotor cortex, from which he derived it. He then trained some of the cats to produce this pattern of brain waves more often by rewarding them with food from an automatic dispenser as soon as the pattern appeared in the EEG. It turned out that the SMR waves did in fact shift the cats into a certain state, in which they were awake while at the same time their bodies were relaxed. This was the first time that brain waves were used to produce a target behavior.

However, the therapeutic benefit of this discovery was not discovered until somewhat later. Sterman was commissioned by NASA to investigate the effect of monomethyl hydrazine, a chemical contained in rocket fuel. It was suspected that even small amounts of this substance impaired astronauts' functional capacities. Sterman therefore tested it in his laboratory cats and found that almost all of them had an epileptic fit one hour after being administered a certain dose of the chemical. However, one group of cats showed a different reaction. They either did not have a fit at all, or it didn't occur until after a considerable delay. And these were the cats whose brains had been trained to produce more SMR frequencies.

One of Barry Sterman's laboratory assistants was particularly fascinated by this result because she herself suffered from epilepsy. Like the cats before her, she also learned to shift her brain into the SMR state more frequently. (Unlike the cats she probably didn't get treats for doing so!) Her efforts were rewarded: she did in fact manage to markedly reduce the number of fits she was having. This experiment that she performed on herself can be considered to mark the start of neurofeedback.

More epilepsy patients were then treated with the neurofeedback method that Sterman had developed (frequency band training), and more positive effects were noticed. Sleep problems disappeared, and in the long term, research subjects who were restless or even hyperactive became calmer. They were able to concentrate better on their everyday activities and their coordination improved. As a result of these discoveries, treatments of sleep disturbances and ADHD became new major fields of application of neurofeedback.

Therapy without a couch or pills

So neurofeedback is by no means a recent discovery, and its results were impressive right from the start. However, it is only recently that it has slowly started to receive the attention that it deserves. One of the reasons for this is no doubt that the number of people who suffer from mental health problems and functional disturbances of the brain is now extremely high. According to a recent study entitled "Study on the Health of Adults in Germany"[1] which was commissioned by the German Federal Health Ministry and published by the Robert Koch Institute, within a period of only a single year one third (!) of the German population was diagnosed with depression, anxiety, addiction, an eating disorder or post-traumatic stress disorder. The study only included cases with full diagnosis.

In 2019 the Global Burden of Disease study reported that 12% of the world's adult population experienced mental illness. In addition to

---

1   Ger: Studie zur Gesundheit Erwachsener in Deutschland (DEGS)

that, in 2020 there was a 28% increase in anxiety and depressive disorders as a result of Covid-19. This increase was higher for women than for men.

The results of an ongoing official study on children's health, the "Children's Health Study"[2] are also worrying. According to its findings, a fifth of 3 to 17-year-olds in Germany have a mental disorder or are at risk of developing one. No fewer than five per cent of children have AD(H)D alone, while a further five per cent have suspected AD(H)D. What is not clear in regard to these figures is whether there really are more cases of ADHD today than in past decades, or whether doctors and patients are simply more aware of it. What we can probably consider certain is that people are now more willing to talk about mental health problems and seek help for them.

The consistently high number of people suffering from mental disorders also indicate that psychotropic drugs are not as effective as expected. However, for a long time they indirectly delayed the wider use of neurofeedback, because swallowing a pill seemed to be a faster and easier way to manage unpleasant states. So many people hoped to obtain relief from pills that the Rolling Stones even dedicated one of their songs, "Mother's little helper" (i.e. tranquilizers), to the issue. But it has now become apparent that medications do not provide sustainable relief from chronic disorders and that they have side effects that can be unpleasant. However, many people have strong reservations about doing psychotherapy or are deterred by the wide choice of different forms of psychotherapy and how long it takes to find a psychotherapist who can offer a free space.

---

2   Ger: Kindergesundheitsstudie (KiGGS)

In their sometimes desperate search for the right treatment people with mental health problems or their families usually hear about neurofeedback by word of mouth. As a method neurofeedback has improved substantially since its beginnings. With the low-frequency trainings (SCP and ILF), which are the methods that have become most widespread, a number of disorders can now be treated at a much deeper level, leading to greater positive effects for clients. The news of these successes spreads. The fact that it is not necessary to start stirring up old stuff that is often painful makes brain training more attractive than psychotherapy for many people – particularly because quite a few have already done psychotherapy, sometimes more than once. In initial consultations I often hear people say things like "I've really had enough of going back over all that again and again", irrespective of whether they mean old childhood experiences, feeling overwhelmed at work or something quite different. Neurofeedback can in fact be a good alternative to psychotherapy, but the optimal solution may also be to combine the two.

It would also be a mistake to believe that it is not necessary to talk at all during neurofeedback. For brain training to be really effective, and particularly with ILF training, the therapist must constantly keep ensuring that they have as accurate a picture of the client's various symptoms as possible. However, most people find it easier to describe sleep disturbances, noises in their ears or headaches than to say why they are not in a good place mentally at the moment. Some people would probably also not be able to say exactly what it is that is causing their depression, anxiety or obsessive-compulsive behavior.

However, it is important for clients to tell their therapist about any previous traumatic experiences, because neurofeedback can open up the doors to our inner junk rooms again and reactivate faded memories.

Neurofeedback should only be used in clients with such problems if the therapist is also well trained in the treatment of psychological traumatization (for more on this see Chapter 7 of Part 3). However, there are no real contra-indications (circumstances in which neuro-feedback may not be used at all), as long as the therapist is well-versed in the disorder(s) from which the client is suffering. With many symptoms it is simply a cost-benefit question as to whether targeted brain training or some other approach is the treatment of choice.

Tracking the symptoms

When people consult me in my office I am only marginally interested in knowing whether they have already been diagnosed, because the boundaries between the various disorders are only rarely clearly demarcated. For instance, some of the children who come with a dia-gnosis of ADHD also have marked autistic traits – and vice versa. Stress, chronic pain, burnout and anxiety are often mixed in ways that vary widely from one person to another. This is not surprising, considering that all of these disorders have a common root, i.e. the fact that the brain's ability to regulate its arousal level is impaired, or never even developed fully in the first place. And that can lead to a broad range of mental and physical symptoms. The symptoms listed on the next few pages will give you an idea of the wide variety of different ways in which an unbalanced brain can draw attention to the fact that it is out of balance.

Symptom checklist

The following list of symptoms provides an overview of the physical and mental phenomena that neurofeedback can have a positive effect on. Many therapists use a list like this to obtain a comprehensive picture of their client's current state and of the changes that occur in the course of the therapy.

General state of health
Exhaustion/tiredness
Frequent infections
Restlessness, tension

Mental performance
Ability to concentrate
Distractibility
Memory
Difficulties with reading
Difficulties with writing
Difficulties with arithmetic
Sense of direction

Emotions
Impulsivity
Mood swings
Anxiety
Anger or aggression
Low mood
Obsessive-compulsive behavior
Risk-taking behavior

Sleep

Difficulty falling asleep

Lying awake at night

Difficulty waking up

Restless sleep

Sleepwalking or night terrors

Nightmares

Clenching or grinding the teeth

Other sleep problems

Digestion

Poor appetite

Excessive appetite (ravenous hunger)

Excessive thirst

Stomach pains

Gut pains (e.g. from gas)

Constipation

Diarrhea

Nausea or vomiting

Irritable bowel

Sensitivity to sugar (e.g. restlessness after consuming foods that contain sugar)

Cardiovascular circulation and respiration

Breathing difficulties

Asthmatic symptoms

High blood pressure

Palpitations/tachycardia (rapid heartbeat)

Pressure in the chest

Disturbances of perception

Double vision

Blurred vision

Pain in the eyes or sensitive eyes

Other eye problems

Hearing loss

Noises in the ears

Sound distortions

Earache

Changes in the sense of smell

Changes in taste

Paresthesias/sensory disturbances (e.g. tingling in the skin)

Lack of sensation in the skin

Hypersensitivity to heat or cold

Pain

Low pain threshold

High pain threshold

Pain that is not so bad, but chronic, or joint stiffness

Chronic, agonizing pain

Chronic nerve pain (burning or sharp)

Headaches

Neurological disorders

Speech problems

Tremor

Movement disorders

Muscle weakness

Disturbances of balance

Difficulties with coordination

Clumsiness or proneness to accidents and injuries

Tics (uncontrollable outbursts of certain speech or movement patterns)

Fainting/loss of consciousness (syncope)

Seizures / Epilepsy

Other

Diabetes

Thyroid disorders

Allergies

Skin problems (e.g. eczema)

Incontinence (in children also bed-wetting)

Premenstrual complaints (Premenstrual Syndrome, PMS)

Menopausal complaints

Addictive behavior

ILF therapists will go through a comprehensive checklist like this item by item, especially at the start of the treatment. This enables them to catch phenomena that the clients themselves would not have thought worth mentioning. It is surprising how often people simply put up with unpleasant symptoms because they know no differently. "That's just how I am", they think, and have no idea that they, too, can be free of constipation or have a restful night's sleep. Hendrik's case is a typical example.

Case example: Insomnia

Hendrik[3] too can sleep!

Hendrik actually consulted me for learning difficulties. He had just turned 15 and had dropped out of school because he couldn't keep up in class. His family was very loving and supported him patiently, but Hendrik simply couldn't concentrate. As always, I asked about all of his symptoms before starting the treatment. He told me that he slept badly and that he almost always needed at least an hour to fall asleep, but neither he nor his parents saw this as a problem. They said tolerantly, "That's just Hendrik" and would have glossed over it. After all, it was his concentration problems they'd come for. When I asked him after three sessions how his sleep was going, Hendrik said happily, "I fall asleep almost before my head touches the pillow!" He was astounded by this development – previously he had never believed that it would be possible for him to sleep well.

As a therapist it is also important for me to know how the client is feeling in as much detail as possible as the treatment goes on. I need these details in order to know which training parameters to use. This applies both to the positioning of the electrodes and to the settings for the feedback signals. How long it takes for the effects to make themselves felt varies. Some people feel so much straight away while the session is still ongoing that I can try out several different settings and have the client train with those that are the best at the time. That doesn't work, of course, if the client does not notice any changes until after the session is over. In that case I have to decide on a single setting at every session because it would not otherwise be possible to link the settings to the client's current response. But while the reaction times vary from one person to another, as a rule they stay the same for each individual person; whether a person notices a change during the session or straight afterwards, or not until one or at the most two days later, stays the same for them – and probably always will.

The number of sessions required for a neurofeedback therapy also depends on such individual differences, not only on the severity of the disorder. In order to alleviate symptoms fast it is also advisable to keep the gap between sessions short at first and preferably to do two sessions a week. Later the schedule can vary greatly – depending on what the client needs and what works timewise. However, unlike the situation with strength training for muscles, we don't need to continue training our brains with neurofeedback for the rest of our lives. For instance, if somebody has overcome depression and then comes up against a challenging situation again at a later stage in their life, we can support the brain once more with a package of five to ten sessions. Genuine relapses usually only occur if the initial therapy was terminated too early. This is actually not unusual, because some clients quickly decide that the treatment is too demanding as soon as they note a substantial improvement.

From all this we can see the extent to which neurofeedback, and especially ILF therapy, are tailored to the needs of the individual client. For this reason the treatments we use for the various disorders and disturbances can only be oriented towards clinical experience of what the treatment could look like, and never conducted according to a fixed "schedule". Even if two people have received the same diagnosis or show similar symptoms, their treatment processes can be completely different!

1. ADD/ADHD: ATTENTION DEFICIT (AND HYPERACTIVITY) DISORDER

This diagnosis covers a whole cluster of symptoms and each person has their own individual mixture of these symptoms. Extreme dreaminess and "spacing or zoning out" are typical of the concentration difficulties in ADD. In contrast, AD-*H*-D is characterized mainly by hyperactivity, i.e. by a strong urge to move, restlessness and erratic behavior.

> Recent studies show that 5 to 10% of children and around 3% of adults worldwide suffer from AD(H)D.

Many children with AD(H)D also lack a good clear sense of their own bodies and therefore appear clumsy or even rough. Their impulse control is also under-developed, which means that they are only rarely able to delay fulfilling their needs and immediately act out all their inner urges. Although this is typical of both forms of the disorder, it gives a bad impression especially in the "explosive", hyperactive variant because it all too often results in behaviors that other people find extremely rude. People with this type of attention deficit disorder therefore rarely receive positive feedback. More often they are admonished and reprimanded, and also ostracized by other people – including other children. But someone who frequently experiences themselves as "wrong" and a failure will not be able to develop a stable sense of self-confidence. Some children are so hurt and sad that they become either depressed or extremely unruly (professionals describe their behavior as "oppositional"). They always have to be antagonistic, and react aggressively and throw tantrums at the slightest provocation.

Adults with ADHD also have difficulty in keeping their temper and not letting their full anger and frustration out on their relatives, friends, colleagues and superiors. They often say and do things that are inexcusable and can have a devastating effect on their relationships.

But what causes this disorder? Dopamine is a neurotransmitter which plays an important role in the brain. It enables impulses to be translated into action, while the frontal lobe decides whether to actually act or not. Remember, the frontal lobe lies behind the forehead (see Part 1, Chapter 1) and takes the longest to mature in the course of child development. It is also particularly prone to disturbances, which can, for instance, result from stressful experiences during childhood, negative family dynamics and poor nutrition. The consumption of large amounts of sugar and many food colorants and other additives and also a deficiency of omega-3 fatty acids (see box) appear to be particularly problematic.

Omega-3 fatty acids for the brain

Scientific findings have long indicated that omega-3 fatty acids are indispensable for brain function and mental stability in all age groups. Children become more intelligent if their mothers have high enough levels of omega-3 fatty acids during pregnancy, and AD(H)D, depression and dementia occur less frequently if there is a high enough intake. In some cases these illnesses may even be alleviated by omega-3 fatty acids if the patient has a severe deficiency and it is rectified. Many people have already heard of these "miraculous" fatty acids, but often do not know how to make use of this information. Doctors are also usually not well-informed about them. If you want to ensure that you yourself or your family are getting enough of these fatty acids, there are some facts that you should be aware of.

Two types of omega-3 fatty acids are active in the body. They have complicated names which are abbreviated to DHA and EPA. To establish whether the tissue level of these substances is high enough the fatty acid profile of the red blood cells is measured. Since these blood cells have a life cycle of about four months, the profile provides a basis for an estimate that is valid for this period. The value obtained is called the omega index and should ideally be somewhere between eight and eleven per cent. On no account should it fall below four per cent. However, research has shown that most people are far too close to this lower limit and hardly anybody manages to reach ideal levels.

How much DHA and EPA is required to reach levels higher than eight per cent varies from one person to another, but, as a guideline, not less than one gram of a mixture of the two types of omega-3 fatty acids are needed daily. Fatty acids are found only in cold water sea fish (which means that fish from the Mediterranean don't count). You would need to eat between 50 g (of herrings) and 200 g (of salmon or mackerel) daily to reach the recommended minimum intake. Fish from aquacultures are often fed large amounts of cereal and therefore contain less DHA and EPA.

If you want to take the fish oil that you can buy in bottles or capsules, you should read the ingredients listed in the small print carefully. How much of the product do you need to take in order to actually take in one gram of the omega-3 fatty acids? If you take that into account, the difference between dietary supplements containing omega 3 that appear to be cheaper and those that seem more expensive often balances out.

Vegetable oils with a high omega-3 content are unfortunately not a real alternative – even if claims are frequently made to the contrary. Only very little of alpha linolenic acid, the vegetable form of the omega-3 fatty acids, is metabolized into the forms that are active in the body. The only non-animal sources of DHA and EPA are certain kinds of micro-algae that are cultured in sea-water tanks, the oil from which is obtainable in the form of food additives.

To date no studies have been conducted on the question as to whether it would have an effect on the neurofeedback treatment if clients were simultaneously to optimize their omega-3 fatty acid levels. I have also not yet heard of anybody trying this in practice, but it could be interesting to follow it up.

However, most experts consider that these factors merely exacerbate the real cause. Experts are in agreement that there is such a thing as an innate predisposition to AD(H)D, but that it tends to develop especially in an environment where there is sensory overload. This can be, for example, chain rattles hanging over babies' diaper changing tables, televisions constantly running, and no escape from the noise of traffic and canned music or flickering neon signs. Children who develop AD(H)D probably have a dysregulation of the dopamine system from birth, which may be either genetic or due to exposure to various influences during pregnancy, e.g. severe mental stress in the mother. Such children then react more strongly to stimulation, which keeps reinforcing this sensitivity.

Boys are especially likely to act out this sensitivity to stimuli – in a way that is still completely uninhibited – and they therefore more often attract negative attention than girls. When girls drift off into a quiet dreaminess, at first glance they appear to be shy, but they also tend to be seen as nice and well-behaved. It is not clear whether boys actually do have AD(H)D more often than girls, or whether the figures are biased due to the differences mentioned above. At all events, boys are diagnosed with AD(H)D almost twice as often as girls. It used to be thought that these children "grow out" of the disorder, but about 60% of them evidently do not. The hyperactivity usually changes into a constant inner restlessness.

Attention deficit disorder is usually treated with various forms of behavioral therapy, often in combination with medications containing the active ingredient methylphenidate, which are better known by their brand names, e.g. Ritalin and Concerta. The greatest objection to these medications is that they have strong side effects and that the desired effects are not sustainable. The old symptoms return as soon as the tablets are discontinued. Some children also sometimes feel very ashamed that other people can only put up with them if they take pills.

AD(H)D and neurofeedback
From the standpoint of neurofeedback AD(H)D is due to reduced levels of brain activation. I like to explain this to clients and their relatives by showing them a simple drawing of the arousal-performance curve (see box). In ADHD sufferers the peak is shifted to the right, and the left side of the curve is much flatter. This means that people with ADHD need

a lot of stimulation to raise their level of arousal to a range in which performance is possible at all. This is also why methylphenidate – a stimulant! – is effective in this disorder. While this seems logical for the "dreamers" and "dawdlers", you will probably find it surprising if you have ever experienced a hyperactive child in action. However, all the restlessness and fidgeting are unconscious strategies the child uses to avoid allowing their attention to wander, and to remain receptive and capable of acting. For these people, doing several things at once and, for example, playing around on their phones during a lecture or a meeting, is like self-therapy. They are *not capable* of being attentive if they are not permitted to do something else at the same time. However, for those in their environment whose brains function differently, this is difficult to accept.

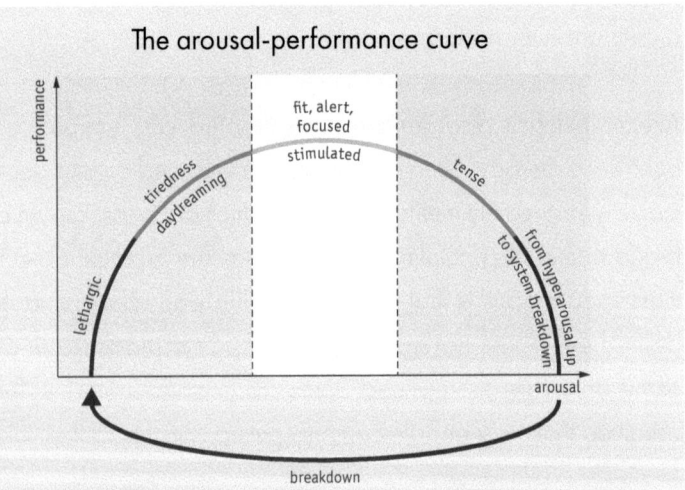

This simple diagram can be drawn on a piece of paper with just a few strokes of the pen and shows clearly how the two parameters arousal and performance are linked. Remember the electric circuit experiments you used to do at school? If the tension is too low, nothing happens, or the light produced in the bulb is only dim, at the most. If it's too high, the system is overloaded and rapidly short circuits. Only when the "juice" in the circuit is correctly regulated are we rewarded with a bright light. If we apply this to the brain's performance capacity, we can say that when the arousal level is too low the person is slow to get going, even when concentrated thinking and goal-directed action are required. But if it is too high, the nervous system reacts sensitively to stimuli and becomes exhausted more quickly. The brain's performance capacity is highest in the medium range, which is shown as lighter area in this diagram. The brain is highly stimulated, and at the same time fresh enough to be able to concentrate well on a task. However, that does not mean that we must busy ourselves with mental challenges during this period – the brain will not rev up like a racing car out of gear if we don't. One can also simply enjoy this state during an evening stroll, without being task-oriented in the classical sense of the term.

If the arousal is lower and the person is relaxed, they experience a pleasant, dreamy state. However, at an even lower arousal level the person is so lethargic that hardly any goal-directed activity is possible. If the brain is well regulated, that is simply the point at which it needs to regenerate itself in restful sleep.

On the other hand, the brain can also be too highly aroused to be able to function in a really optimal way. It slips into this tense state when it has to handle a large number of stimuli without sufficient rest periods. While it is still possible to get a lot done in such a state, it is more of an effort than should in fact be necessary. Moreover, it becomes less and less likely that it will be possible to accomplish tasks that require foresight and creativity. If the hyperarousal increases even further, this is experienced as an existential threat that can only be coped with by fighting, fleeing or freezing completely (playing dead). The arrow at the bottom shows symbolically that such a situation leads to severe exhaustion. In burnout states this is so severe and all-encompassing that sufferers are catapulted into the tense or hyperaroused range by even the smallest challenge.

In all functional disturbances of the brain that occur in the form of attacks (in neurofeedback these are called "instabilities") the whole graph is much narrower. People who experience such attacks not only slip out of the optimal state more easily, but the consequences are often also extreme and can result in panic attacks, migraine or epileptic seizures, for instance.

Interestingly, in some situations this property of the brain can also be an advantage. For example, I once ran a sailing course where there was a participant who nearly always appeared to be absent-minded and drove everybody crazy with his slow reaction times. But one day we got caught in a storm and suddenly Peter was in his element – whereas the other beginners were rather overwhelmed. When sailing in normal weather they had been able to carry out all the procedures correctly and promptly, but they were unable to do so in a situation where the conditions changed much faster than they were accustomed to and they were bombarded with stimuli. Peter, however, came into his own and worked with a determination and speed that surprised everyone – including me. Although as a therapist I am familiar with such phenomena, I am still often amazed when I experience them outside the consulting room.

However, ideally we should be able to remain focused and react appropriately when less activity is required. It is precisely this ability that is developed through neurofeedback. In order to find the right training parameters I always start by establishing the range of symptoms and then gauge whether to strengthen calming and letting-go tendencies, or activating and controlling tendencies. Thus, for example, impulse control is an active capacity, but it would not be a good idea to train the brain in this direction if the client still showed too strong a tendency towards restlessness. I would like to show what that means in practical terms in the following case example of Justin (I will return to the issue of obsessive-compulsive disorders later on.)

Case example: ADHD (child)
First calm down, then build up strength

When Justin came to me, he was seven years old and had already been diagnosed with ADHD. He was extremely restless, constantly broke things and couldn't stand it when he couldn't get his own way. He was also hardly able to concentrate on anything, but when something did catch his interest, it wasn't possible to prize him off it again. He had to be told everything several times before it really sank in. He had great difficulty with changes. If they were not introduced slowly and explained in detail, he would immediately work himself up into an emotional crisis, lose his temper and scream nonstop.

This combination of symptoms led me to suspect that Justin was probably also suffering from Asperger's syndrome, i.e. a form of autism. This was also indicated by the fact that he was unable to look other people in the eye and was far ahead of his peers in some areas. For instance, he learned to read at an early age, had an extremely good memory and understood complicated scientific facts about astrophysics.

Because he was so restless and emotionally unstable I began the neurofeedback training in a way that strengthens the brain's calming capacities. One thing that was very helpful in finding the right feedback for him was that he would keep shutting his eyes tightly in a characteristic way. This kind of behavior is called a tic. Some settings reinforced this behavior, while others immediately reduced it substantially.

The first treatment successes occurred after only three sessions – so fast that Justin's family could hardly keep up with them. Surprised, his father said, "All of a sudden we don't have to repeat everything a hundred times before he gets it." In my office, too, I observed a marked change. Now when Justin came he would still scurry around for a while before he sat down, but his actions were goal-oriented and constructive. For instance, he would straighten his chair and fetch a blanket and the cuddly toy. He was also quite soon able to hold his gaze, so the darting around of his eyes had only been due to his agitation. His father also reported that his emotional crises had become much less frequent and dramatic, and that it no longer took so long to calm Justin down. However, at some point I received the feedback that he had started to pull at his hair again. He would rub small strands of it into knots and sometimes even pull them out. That was an important indication for me that I should shift the direction of his treatment. In order to be able to break bad habits you need control, and that is an active ability. If a child pulls their hair it is a clear indication that the therapy needs to be adjusted accordingly, to strengthen their capacity to control their impulses.

However, people with ADHD typically also have the problem that they are not at all aware of the state of arousal they are currently in. They think they feel equally good all the time and make only few useful comments even when I make greater changes to the feedback settings. For many people who have disorders that occur in the form of attacks, the effect of that would be unbearable! However, once we have found the right parameters for them, they often experience positive effects in their daily lives quite soon. With Justin, for example, that happened after only three sessions. It is always a wonderful moment when a child reports new experiences with a smile on their face and says, for example, "The others said they can see awesome changes in me." Or, "My teacher told me I am doing well!"

Sometimes this positive attitude collapses again after a while. This is because through the training the clients learn to judge themselves better and realize how many skills they lack. In this phase typical remarks are, for example, "I'm not nearly as good as all the others in my class". Or, "How will I be able to get a job when I've finished school if I don't pass my exams?" In such cases it is important that they have private tuition or professional coaching or do some other supportive activity in addition to the neurofeedback.

What is also not unusual is that the children themselves make good progress, and yet their family or classmates and teacher don't really notice. Then I sometimes have them do a "Continuous Performance Test" (see Part 2, Chapter 3) so that their parents can see from the improvement in their ability to concentrate what progress their child has already made. However, sometimes it is necessary for the parents to do extra family counseling to help the family to find a really good way of getting along with each other. However, it not infrequently happens that one or other parent realizes that they themselves have

AD(H)D and that it's not only due to the child that the family harmony is constantly disturbed. This happened in the case of Michael. Read his own description of his case below.

Case example: ADHD (adult)
My impulsivity got me into lot of trouble

I only discovered that I have ADHD twelve years ago – when I was 36. A teacher spoke to me and my wife about our son's behavior and everything she described seemed very familiar to me. It sounded like the story of my own schooldays. I consulted a psychologist who confirmed my suspicions. When I was a child nobody knew anything about this disorder, people would just say, "That's just how he is." I was impulsive, restless and wild, but I could also really space out when things were boring – and at school that was unfortunately most of the time.

I really suffered a lot at school and in the end it took me 13 years to get the school-leaving certificate that other people get when they're 15. I was constantly being told that I was lazy or didn't make enough effort. Only one teacher recognized that I was actually capable of doing well. I would often get sick before a class test – really sick, I wasn't faking it. And when I had to do the test later, this teacher would often "forget" that I was there, and so I would be able to go on writing for another half an hour. That helped me tremendously. Later I did the entrance exam for universities of applied science and studied for a degree. It is in fact surprising that I have made a career for myself in spite of everything. Probably because I was intelligent enough to always somehow muddle through, but also because my family supported me.

My parents are very tolerant and gave me a lot of space, I was lucky there. And it was also my salvation, because when I left school at 19 and was doing odd jobs, I really went off the rails – experimented with drugs and stuff. At some point my parents and my siblings gave me a talking to and asked me, "What are you doing? Where do you think this is going to lead?" And then I got my act together.

But it's mainly my impulsivity that has really been damaging at work, again and again. More than once I've told a boss straight what I think of his decisions – and not everyone can take that. With one of them it was really bad, we just didn't hit it off and were constantly fighting. He would trigger something in me so strongly that I would often really lose it. I'm sure it was only because my parents were so tolerant that my impulsivity didn't end in violent outbursts.

When both I and my children were diagnosed with ADHD I did some research on the internet and finally came across neurofeedback. Seven years ago all of us did the therapy with Meike Wiedemann. At about 30 sessions per person it cost quite a lot of money – I even took out a loan to pay for it – but it was worth it. It helped me enormously. I haven't become a different person, but I've got a handle on my impulsivity – even with the one boss who gets on my nerves so much. And now I also find it much easier to concentrate on things that are rather boring. With my son it's also made his impulsivity controllable, today he's very even-tempered. The therapy hasn't made him much keener to go to school, but I'm sure he'll find a path for himself, anyway. His sister has benefited more in that direction, she likes to learn, in fact, and is able to concentrate better now.

What I am especially pleased about is that our family life used to be really stressful, with screaming, slamming doors and stuff, really awful.

Today my children like hanging out with me and I with them. And that's really great.

2. AUTISM SPECTRUM DISORDER (ASD) / ASPERGER'S SYNDROME

The issue of autism was probably first brought into public awareness in 1988 by the movie "Rain Man". Dustin Hoffman even got an Oscar for his performance of Raymond, a man with autism. At that time this severe developmental disorder had only been known to professionals for about 40 years, although it is by no means rare. According to current estimates, roughly one out of 100 children suffer from autism, if we include the whole spectrum of different forms in which it can occur. In some cases the diagnosis is not made until adulthood.

Two doctors were the first to describe autism, independently of each other. Surprisingly, both of them, Leo Kanner, an American psychiatrist, and Hans Asperger, an Austrian pediatrician, gave the cluster of phenomena they observed the same name: autism. Their intention was to draw attention to the fact that the disorder was mainly a disturbance of contact: people with autism are typically withdrawn and inaccessible to other people, and have great difficulty in connecting with other people. They register and process sensory impressions such as light, sounds and touch differently from healthy people and rapidly experience them as stressful or even unbearable.

However, autistic disorders can vary substantially in severity. At one end of the spectrum there are those who may perhaps appear somewhat eccentric, but are able to lead a relatively normal life that includes doing some sort of training, holding down a job and having a family and children. At the other end there are people whose impairments are so severe that they need an enormous amount of support all their lives. The milder forms of autism are sometimes also called "Asperger's syndrome", but many specialists now no longer use this term. The symptoms of the two disorders evidently overlap more than was originally thought and they cannot be clearly distinguished from one another.

The common thread running through all the different forms is that the person has little or no feeling for another person's inner life and has great difficulty in putting themselves in someone else's shoes. But we need this capacity in order to be able to communicate with other people, understand their feelings and orient ourselves within a community.

Whereas for healthy people decoding body language is as natural as breathing, people with autism have great difficulty in doing so. Some of them manage to understand other people's behavior by interpreting it by means of a process of logical reasoning. In other words, they have learned by heart what people typically do in certain situations and how one should then react – as if they were interacting with a person from another tribe or even from a completely different species. But even if that works, they usually remain unable to grasp jokes, plays on words told with a wink or irony, because they take them literally.

It is possible that in autistic people even their ability to relate to their own self is disturbed. At least, that is what we can assume from the reports of Temple Grandin, a well-known autistic person who has managed to work her way far enough out of the disorder to describe it in books and lectures. Autistic people's thinking is often very concrete, and has little of the subjectivity and emotionality that is quite normal for most people. In contrast, their thinking seems more like data processing (Grandin actually does often use technical terms to describe it) – it lacks liveliness, is rigid and process-like, but on the other hand very precise in certain domains. Like many "high-functioning" autistic people, Grandin is highly intelligent and has amazing talents.

People with autism also very typically dedicate themselves almost obsessively to a narrowly defined field of interest. However, what fascinates outsiders are what are known as savant skills, abilities that seem almost supernatural in a person who is otherwise unable to master things that even toddlers can do. For instance, in the movie mentioned above, Raymond learns a fat telephone directory off by heart and needs only to glance at a pile of toothpicks that have fallen on the floor to know that there are 246 of them. To give an example from real life, Stephen Wiltshire is able to make highly detailed drawings of a town that he has seen only once during a sightseeing flight. On his website www.stephenwiltshire. co.uk you will find a link to an impressive video that shows him drawing. No less than ten per cent of autistic people are in the group of "savants", as people with such out-of-the-ordinary capacities are called.

The typical negative symptoms of autism include hypersensitivity and being unable to tolerate even the smallest changes. Even something like being given a new toothbrush or having to get into a car in a different way from usual can trigger a severe emotional crisis or a screaming fit. Autistic people can be completely riveted by things and activities that seem senseless, such as turning a stone round and round. They may also have a wide variety of tics, i.e. stereotypical movements, and disturbances of coordination and speech abnormalities. The latter range from a strangely formulaic, toneless way of speaking to repeating senseless sentences.

Autism may be due to a genetic predisposition, and also to problems arising during pregnancy, environmental influences, metabolic disorders or inflammation of the brain. It is four times more frequent in boys than in girls. Whether that has to do with male hormones or is genetically determined, or whether it is simply diagnosed more often, is a matter of debate. To date there is neither a psychotherapeutic nor a medical treatment for autism.

Autism and neurofeedback

In clinical practice autism and AD(H)D are often closely interwoven. This is likely because in both cases there is a dysfunction of the sentinel and resting state networks. As described above in Section 1, the resting state network needs to be active in order for us to be able to process impressions and experiences and develop a personal stance towards them. This is where we link the way we perceive the world, how we relate to it and how we find our place within it as an individual. The theory that the resting state network fails to "start" would explain why people with autism also have difficulty in getting in touch with their own inner processes – and without this consciousness of self, contact with other people also remains blocked.

It is not so long ago that people with autism were prescribed stimulants because it was believed that they were unreceptive to stimuli. And yet it is the other way round: autistic people are extremely hyper-sensitive because they lack the capacity to weigh impressions against each other. In the classroom autistic children experience everything with equal intensity – the noise of the traffic outside the window, the shadows that the swaying of the leaves in the wind project on to the wall, the brightly colored sweater of the child sitting next to them, and somewhere in this flood of impressions also what the teacher is saying. This is why they are so insistent that everything must stay the same: stable structures make the constant input more bearable. Other strategies they use are withdrawing from social situations, seeking environments that are as low in stimulation as possible and withdrawing into total inner isolation.

The hyperarousal of the brain disrupts the functioning mainly of the "emotional" right brain hemisphere, while in the analytical left hemisphere it can lead to exceptional performance; however, the achievements remain rigidly restricted to certain channels. For example, an autistic person may be able to learn an entire bus timetable by heart, but that doesn't help them if their bus doesn't arrive at exactly 8.32. Due to the extreme excitability of their brains they are completely disconcerted by even the smallest deviation – their thought processes are narrowed as if they were in a situation of existential threat, although they in fact know when the next bus should leave.

In ILF training the initial goal is therefore to calm the right brain hemisphere. The great advantage of this form of neurofeedback lies in the fact that it can be used to treat even very small children and children with severe delays in their development. New behaviors become possible as soon as the client's brain learns how to down-regulate the hyperarousal of the right hemisphere. It does, of course, vary from one client to another how long the training takes, but initial successes are usually achieved rapidly. Being able to achieve a marked reduction in the suffering of the clients and their families after only a few sessions makes it very satisfying to work with autistic clients.

How meaningful the treatment successes are for clients and their relatives is best illustrated by a letter from a mother that reached me on my return from a Christmas break. She had previously traveled down to Stuttgart from northern Germany with her son Luca on three occasions so that he could do intensive training, which consisted of a treatment cycle of ten sessions over five days. The boy showed characteristics that were clearly autistic, as well as symptoms of ADHD.

Case example: Autism
The changes in Luca as seen by his family

Dear Meike,
Please forgive me for not having written sooner. I was really skeptical whether Luca's progress would really last. But it has! I don't know how to put into words how grateful I am. He can express himself, speaks in long, complete sentences, asks questions himself and answers questions. He is aware of what is happening around him, is interested in it and comments on it, too. He laughs at jokes and even tries to joke himself!!! His memory has also improved. If you ask him to do something you don't have to repeat it only a few seconds later. He also talks about you and says you helped him, that he likes going to you and that you are cool!

He talks to his schoolmates and can also talk on the phone, without simply repeating what other people say. He evidently understands better what other people are feeling. He is also better able to concentrate on his homework. Wow! Our neighbors are doctors and they are very impressed by how much Luca has changed. I am also hearing only good things about his progress from other people, including some of our friends and his teachers. For example, Luca's class teacher has said that his pronunciation has improved and that he thinks more analytically and arrives at more suitable solutions. He can remember things better and describe what he remembers, and is slowly becoming able to put events in the right order. He can now count and grasp the meaning of numbers. He is also better coordinated and his sense of orientation has improved.

He has also suddenly started to want to play the piano, too! We fetched a piano from his grandparents that was just standing around and got it tuned, now he tinkles around on it every day. We'll see how that develops.

We are so grateful for all of this!!! We will keep you up to date with developments and we'll definitely come to Stuttgart again.

Thanks a million, dear Meike!

Denise, Luca and Martin

3. DEPRESSION – BURNOUT –
BIPOLAR DISORDER

Depression is officially defined as an "affective" disorder and described as an intensely sad, dispirited, completely exhausted state which has lasted for not less than two weeks. People with depression are have no interest in anything and are unable to enjoy anything or bring themselves to do anything. According to the "Study on the Health of Adults in Germany" mentioned above, roughly ten per cent of women and six per cent of men in Germany report having been diagnosed with depression in the past year.[3] However, the authors of the study assume that many more people are suffering from deep despair.

Today it is easy to get the impression that depression is spreading like an epidemic, but it is not clear whether the numbers are really so much higher than they used to be. What is certain is that people are now talking more about depression. That is a good thing, but it must not be trivialized or thought of as a kind of "aggravated bad mood". Depression stifles all pleasure and can make life such a torment that 15 per cent of sufferers see no other option but to commit suicide. According to the official statistics, up to 70 per cent of all suicides are due to depression.

Psychiatrists differentiate between several different forms of depression. In some cases depression simply happens, with no apparent external reason for the low mood. Some psychiatrists refer to this as endogenous depression. In other cases the mood change has clearly

---

3   Globally, an estimated 5% of adults suffer from depression (WHO).

been preceded by some form of psychological stress. This is also the case with burnout, a state similar to depression, which is triggered by high levels of stress in the workplace. There are no clear dividing lines between depression and burnout. Burnout sufferers typically tend to be perfectionist and to want to please everybody. Unconsciously they adhere to the belief that if things don't go well they need to try even harder.

Winter blues or genuine depression?

Winter often doesn't make it easy for us to stay in a good mood. When we leave the house it is still dark and when we come back home it is dark again. In between it is mainly gray, gloomy, wet and cold. Everything seems to reject us: people withdraw into their homes or wrap themselves up in thick coats. But while at this time of year some people are able to find fuel for their gallows humor on even the most horrible damp day, and look forward to a cup of tea, candles and the sauna, other people feel down in the dumps for weeks or even months. If you feel like that too, you have probably wondered whether you are in fact depressed.

In fact, there is no clear dividing line between "winter blues" and an illness that is serious enough to require treatment. If severe, this kind of illness may be diagnosed as "Seasonal Affective Disorder", which is abbreviated to SAD. Up to a certain point it is normal for our mood to be lower from mid-October onwards than it is in summer. Issues such as farewells, death and emptiness then start to hold sway in nature and few people are able to completely escape the melancholy that this provokes. Against this backdrop, memories of painful experiences and losses are more easily reactivated and problems are perceived as being more serious.

However, it is also simply the lack of light that lowers our mood. The sun is the most important driver of our internal clock. It has the strongest effect on our biorhythm via the neurotransmitter melatonin, for example. The brighter the light, the less the body secretes of this neurotransmitter that makes us sleepy. In twilight the production of melatonin increases, and it reaches its highest point at about 3 o'clock in the morning. If you are awake at that time (and not still dancing at a party) you are usually feeling somewhat out of sorts. You are not really able to handle things, all problems seem enormous, and life as a whole seems tiring, gray and joyless. The similarities to winter blues are not coincidental. It has been found that people who suffer from winter blues also have increased melatonin levels during the day. The fact that this neurotransmitter is produced from serotonin and that the level of serotonin, which is flippantly referred to as a "happy hormone", therefore falls, lowers the mood even further.

While this imbalance in the chemistry of the brain is probably not the only reason for the gloominess, light can still help – often even in severe cases. The most important strategy is to go out into the sun every day if possible, ideally early in the morning. Even on dull days, sunlight is still stronger than the vast majority of artificial lights. Another option is to sit in front of a therapy lamp while having your breakfast. The lamp should have the same light spectrum as the sun and reach at least 10000 lux. However, it can take two weeks before your mood lifts.

Bipolar disorders are a specific form of affective disorder in which the person alternates or "cycles" between depressive and manic states. In mania they are brimming over with energy and embark on high-flying projects. While they themselves usually feel really good during this phase, they are nonetheless at risk. They may injure themselves because they overestimate their physical capacities. Or they may throw all their savings out of the window or put their very means of existence at risk in an attempt to realize some crazy plan, such as opening a beach bar in the Caribbean. Cyclothymia is also a disorder that involves mood fluctuations, but they are less extreme than in bipolar disorder.

> Depression can also arise as a side effect of medications or concomitantly with other illnesses, such as chronic infections, cancer or hormonal disturbances.

One major factor in the development of all forms of depression is assumed to be a disturbance in the metabolism of neurotransmitters, especially serotonin. However, many experts now reject this explanation, seeing it as an oversimplification that only became popular after the arrival of antidepressants on the market. The active ingredients of the most frequently prescribed antidepressants work by enhancing the effect of the serotonin released at the synapses (see Part 1, Chapter 3). All forms of depression are also treated with psychotherapy and body therapy. Exercise has also been demonstrated to have a positive effect, although the effect is mainly preventive, since few people who are in the middle of a depressive episode will manage to rouse themselves to do any exercise.

One of the most effective short-acting treatments is sleep deprivation. Many of those who try it feel much better and considerably more productive after a night without any sleep. However, it is unclear why this is so. Unfortunately the effect only lasts for one day, but that can be decisive in giving the person the strength to get help.

In severe cases that do not respond to other treatment methods, doctors are now increasingly beginning to fall back on various forms of electrical stimulation. In electroconvulsive therapy (ECT) an electric current is passed through certain areas of the brain in order to trigger a seizure. The patient is placed under anesthetic and given medication to ensure that their muscles remain relaxed. No conclusive explanation has yet been found as to why this rather crude procedure helps – my impression is that it simply triggers a kind of "reset" in the brain. How long patients feel better afterwards varies considerably.

In vagus nerve stimulation doctors implant a small pacemaker in the patient which emits weak electrical impulses to the "control center" for involuntary bodily functions. Here again there is no generally accepted model that would explain why this improves patients' mood. The same applies to transcranial magnetic stimulation (TMS), which has as yet been mainly employed in experimental contexts. It involves stimulating the brain from outside with strong magnetic waves. The patient feels only a tingling sensation in the scalp.

To me it is not at all surprising that such externally applied impulses stimulate the brain to reorganize itself. However, this can often be achieved more effectively with neurofeedback because the training always reflects back what it is doing directly – and that enhances the learning effect.

Depressive disorders and neurofeedback

In depression it is also the case that the arousal level of the brain has become disrupted – but contrary to what one might suppose, it is often too high. While people with depression have no drive and are listless, they are also extremely tense, restless, and full of anxiety and despair. They are therefore unable to "get their act together", as they themselves often put it, because they are so totally exhausted. In this state even taking the garbage out can feel like an impossible feat. This also makes it easier to understand bipolar disorder: sometimes the arousal level tips in one direction and sometimes in the other.

> As the thyroid gland has a strong influence on our inner arousal level, before starting neurofeedback therapy it should be established whether it is working well or whether it needs support from medication. That is particularly true in depression, but also applies in many of the other disorders described in this book.

As the following case example with Daniel shows, neurofeedback therapy is also effective in forms of depression where no external cause is evident. However, it is a laborious procedure – it takes time.

Case example: Depression with no apparent external cause
And then we're back at square one

Daniel had always had a tendency to be feel low. He was now 23 and there was still no evidence of any causes or triggers of his depressions, nor had any been found when he was in psychotherapy. While he was at university his condition deteriorated so much that he had to drop out of his studies and return to his parents' care – how humiliating for a young man! He kept his appointments regularly, but was by no means convinced that neurofeedback could help him. One of his most frequent remarks was, "This is all pointless".

The treatment of depression in cases where the patient is not aware of a triggering stressor is often more uphill work than it is with other patients, and the first signs of improvement are often very subtle and tend to be easier for other people to perceive than for the patient themselves. This was also true in Daniel's case. After a few sessions I observed that his gaze was calmer, his voice sounded less flat and what he told me was no longer so incoherent. The next thing was that his parents saw him as being more active at home. But it was only after 13 sessions that he himself noticed that things were getting better. He started to go jogging again, not just to boost his health or have something to do – he really looked forward to running and wanted to get fitter.

The exercise reinforced the upswing that the neurofeedback had set in motion. Daniel positively flourished. He embarked on various projects and even developed some ideas as to how he could turn them into a career. At this point he had had about 20 sessions. As positive as his development was, I was not yet sure that his condition was stable. But he was determined to stop the therapy. Since I cannot (and would not want to) force anyone to do training, I accepted his decision. I did, however, impress on him that he should contact me straight away if his mood should darken again.

He did, in fact, fall into the depths of despair again after one of his projects failed just over a year later, but he did not get in touch. A good friend finally "dragged" him to see me. For me the ensuing treatment was "déjà-vu" from the word go. Once again, Daniel was reluctant to come for his appointments, didn't see the point of the treatment and hardly noticed the initial improvements. I did, of course, remind him of how the previous round of sessions had gone – knowing full well that that rarely helps in such situations. If a person has no drive in their brain, it doesn't usually help them if you say something like, "The last time going jogging really did you good".

Daniel did keep going with this second round of therapy until I was of the opinion that he was really stable. In order not to burn himself out in projects that were doomed to fail, but rather to try to find the right career solution for himself, he also did sessions with a coach specialized in that field.

Where patients are aware of the stress factors that preceded their illness and also in burnout a good way to explain what happens is to show the arousal-performance curve (see Part 3, Chapter 1). Due to their life situations and personal coping strategies people with depression and burnout remain stuck in a state of tense tiredness for long periods – sometimes even for years – and keep slipping into the red area at the bottom. Breakdown can come very suddenly if an additional weight is added when the burden is already too heavy – all at once the person's strength is completely exhausted.

A process like this is typical of burnout. The treatment can sometimes be very long and drawn-out because the clients present with such an "inner vibration" that they experience even the mildest training parameters as unbearably strong. With one client I finally had to fall back on a DVD with a film of an aquarium that had been shot with a single camera setting. Even an animated cartoon of an aquarium was too stressful for her. It takes a long time for these clients to get back on their feet. They have depleted their resources so thoroughly that there's nothing left to activate – and they have to build up their strength again from rock bottom in a slow and difficult process. In cases like this, neurofeedback training should always be combined with psychotherapy or coaching, in order to find new ways of coping with demands.

The treatment is considerably easier if the clients are in total breakdown when they arrive for their appointment – as was Bernd. Neurofeedback didn't solve his problem, but it did help him to shift into more restorative states and thus remain able to act.

Case example: Depression with a discernible triggering stress factor
When the burden simply gets too great

Bernd (45) is a typical high-functioning guy. He works very hard at his job and is highly successful. But one day his wife suddenly became severely psychotic. In his eyes she was endangering herself and other people (not least their children), but he couldn't find anybody who would really listen to him. The stress associated with this situation gradually sapped all his strength and he finally became completely exhausted.

It is in fact very stressful when things remain unresolved and there is nothing one can do about it. People with this problem often feel left hanging in the air and simply don't know how to handle their anger, despair and grief. This was different from Bernd's work problems, where he would simply deal with the problem by leaving – here he could not do that, since it would mean leaving his children.

Bernd came for neurofeedback because his sleep was severely disturbed, he had no energy and was constantly irritated by his staff and his children. "Before, I would have forgotten a strenuous phase after a weekend, but now I can't even recharge my batteries in a week's vacation", he said. If he could have, he would have withdrawn to a lonely island where he wouldn't have to see anybody or do anything. He refused to do psychotherapy, "that's just blathering, it doesn't do any good". But not only did he not mind answering questions about his symptoms for the neurofeedback treatment, he was also particularly good at describing how each of the different settings felt for him during a session.

To start with Bernd came twice a week. Immediately after the first session he had the feeling that "the layers of the onion are opening up". He soon started to sleep better, which is always good for recovery. Immediately after the sessions he would feel relaxed for a prolonged period and had a less gloomy outlook on the world. However, in one session the feedback parameters were not well adjusted, and this plunged him into a depressive phase. That was, of course, a setback that can always happen. However, such effects can be reversed in the next session by going back to settings that worked better. That also worked with Bernd – luckily the setback did not shake his confidence in me or the method.

At the end of the treatment he still had not been able to solve his problems, but his "tunnel vision" had opened up. He was able to see ways in which the situation might still be changed and experienced himself as being capable of acting. He was also better able to cope with everyday challenges and no longer felt crushed by them.

I often receive inquiries from people who have to travel a long way to come and see me and would therefore like to do intensive training. However, if they are depressed I will not do that if the patient intends to come to Stuttgart on their own, since, as with all treatments of depression, with neurofeedback the lack of drive may subside first, while the low mood still persists. For some patients this would remove the only brake that prevents them from committing suicide. It is therefore imperative that the therapist mention this uncomfortable issue and ensure that the client is accompanied by somebody else at the start of the training – e.g. a family member, a friend or, if no-one else is available, a member of staff from a clinic.

4. ANXIETY DISORDERS

From a biological point of view fear is the reaction to the feeling of being under threat. It is not always that easy to evaluate whether this fear is "appropriate". However, it needs to be treated at the latest when it results in inordinate restrictions in our lives. According to the World Health Organization an estimated 4% of the global population currently experience anxiety disorder. In 2019, 301 million people in the word had an anxiety disorder, making anxiety disorders the most common of all mental disorders.

There is a difference between phobias and general anxiety disorder. With phobias the excessive fears are triggered by specific things such as spiders or occur in specific situations, for example in a crowd. In generalized anxiety disorder there are no such clear causes and yet there is a certain amount of overlap between the two different types.

Typical symptoms of an anxiety attack are a racing heart and/or palpitations, trembling, breaking into a sweat, shortness of breath, dizziness, tightness and pains in the chest, nausea, loss of sensation or tingling in the arms and legs – all the reactions that occur when a person is in a truly life-threatening situation. However, if patients are unable to identify an external cause for their reaction they are convinced that they are physically ill. As a rule their doctor will also follow this up first. If the final diagnosis is some form of "anxiety disorder" – sometimes only after many tests have been done – patients do not necessarily feel relieved. It is hard for them to imagine that such overwhelming symptoms can happen "just like that" and so they remain worried that the doctor might have missed something.

But of course panic attacks and other anxiety disorders don't just come out of the blue. Sometimes they can quite clearly be traced back to a traumatic event – be it an accident, a crime or a natural disaster. In other cases the cause of the apparently totally irrational anxieties is not so easy to identify. It is typical for the patient to experience intense inner tension, the cause of which may lie in a past psychological injury or in acute stress experienced in the present. Examples of the latter might be being under extreme pressure at work, going through a difficult divorce or having all one's strength sapped by caring for a loved one. Often several such factors come together.

> Breathing is decisive in panic attacks. When patients begin to hyperventilate (often without being aware of it) the pH value of the blood changes, which makes the muscles go into spasm. So they are getting themselves into a physical state that can be experienced as extremely dangerous. Therefore if you feel an attack is imminent it helps to focus on consciously exhaling, which counteracts the hyperventilation.

Both the "anticipatory tension" in regard to everything that has to do with what makes the patient anxious, and constant anxious self-observation play a large part in the process. Many people who have experienced panic attacks pay too much attention to every small thing that happens in their body and are literally waiting for the next attack, thus getting caught up in a self-perpetuating cycle. The brain often connects a panic attack with the situation in which it happened, which results in the anxiety being transferred to something completely harmless, such as traveling on the subway, for example. This link can be reinforced if the person feels so unwell during later trips on the subway that they become agitated, which escalates into a new attack. But the link would become closer even if they avoid the subway after that. If a person avoids situations that they perceive as dangerous they may end up hardly daring to leave the house.

Curing phobias fast

There are various quick and easy methods for treating specific phobias such as a fear of spiders or the fear of flying. This does not necessarily involve confronting the person with the very situation that frightens them– this misconception puts many people off even thinking about seeking treatment. If the therapist or coach focuses on the way in which the brain learns an irrational fear and gets more and more worked up about it, they can use the same process to help the client learn to react in a different way. To do this it is essential to direct the client's imagination in a skillful way. You will remember that for the brain it makes hardly any difference whether it is really experiencing something, remembering it or fantasizing the whole scenario. So neuro-linguistic programming (NLP), for example, has developed sophisticated techniques to eliminate phobias fast (which is why these techniques have come to be known as the "Fast Phobia Cure").

What has proved particularly effective is to "feed" the subconscious with new, positive images in trance-like states such as those attained through hypnosis. A therapist with experience in this field can also support this process with neurofeedback (alpha synchrony training) which makes it easier to lead the client into this deeply relaxed and receptive state. Incidentally, there is no reason to be afraid of hypnotic states – the client is by no means "out of it" but awake and always in a position to come out of the trance themselves.

Medication is now no longer the treatment of choice for anxiety disorders, because some of the drugs prescribed, in particular benzodiazepines (which are classed as anxiolytics or sedatives) can be highly addictive. According to the results of the US National Study on Drug-Use and Health published in 2023, an estimated 17.7% of all people who used benzodiazepines reported misusing them in the past year. There are also various plant-based medicines that reduce anxiety and have a calming effect. Although they are not strong enough to treat genuine panic attacks, they can be used to support other therapies. Nowadays we know that body oriented therapies are more successful in improving the patient's situation than talk therapies. The reason is that the fear reaction is rooted in areas of the brain which are hardly accessible to consciousness, but which communicate all the more intensively with the body. The aim is to enable the senses, muscles and nervous system to experience something other than the things that produce fear or anxiety, in other words expansiveness rather than tightness, mobility rather than a frozen state, and relaxation rather than tension. Biofeedback and hypnosis can also help the patient to reduce their inner restlessness and remain calm even in those situations that they find most threatening.

Anxiety disorders and neurofeedback

Neurofeedback can be used to get to the root of the hyperarousal of anxiety patients – at the level of the subconscious. I often design the training in such a way that a marked reduction in bodily tension is achieved at the start of the treatment. The clients then feel better and are able to perceive symptoms such as an erratic heartbeat or breathlessness, which we all experience occasionally, in a detached way. They do not automatically feel threatened by them. Next I select the position of the electrodes in such a way that the clients become more emotionally stable. However, if a person's anxiety is causing obsessive-compulsive thoughts or actions, then different areas of the brain must be trained. The following example of Manfred's treatment shows what the training can look like in practice.

Case example: Anxiety disorder
Getting a hold on anxiety

Manfred (48) had always tended to worry a lot and ruminate about worst-case scenarios, but over the years these fearful thoughts had become more and more persistent. He was most worried that he might have an accident, and first this led to his stopping flying. It later made cycling more and more stressful (he used to cycle to work), and eventually he didn't even want to get into a car. When he came for an appointment with me he was suffering from sleep disturbances and had already experienced several panic attacks that he found extremely frightening, not only as they were happening, but also in regard to his future career prospects. So far he had managed to conceal the attacks but he was afraid that his colleagues were already beginning to talk about it at work.

He already started to sleep much better after the second session, which he found very encouraging. After five sessions I tried out a particular position for the electrodes that often helps to reduce compulsive thoughts. However Manfred responded with a very rapid heartbeat and palpitations. So I switched to other positions which achieved the soothing effect on his thoughts a few sessions later. Over the course of 20 appointments the other anxiety symptoms also gradually subsided and Manfred was again able to use all types of transport. However, he did have another panic attack which came without warning while he was dozing on the sofa. Why that happened is unclear.

Ultimately, however, this setback was good for Manfred's further re-habilitation because it gave him the feeling that he had things under control – he was able to get the attack to subside himself. Afterwards he was still in a fit enough state to do what he had planned for the rest of the day. This experience helped him to get better and better at dealing with slight hints of anxiety. Finally we increased the amount of time between appointments more and more and ended the treatment after 30 sessions.

For me as the therapist it is satisfying when I can tie up a session of treatment so "neatly", but it is not always possible. With Stefanie, another anxiety patient, I was unable to make progress with ILF neurofeedback.

Case example: Anxiety disorder
Stefanie under pressure

Stefanie (38) was actually managing her anxiety problems well by taking medication. However, she wanted to have a baby and didn't want to take any medication during the pregnancy. When she heard about neurofeedback she thought this might provide a way out of the dilemma.

However, the treatment didn't run smoothly right from the start. Stefanie was one of those people who plan everything very precisely and want to stay in control. She fired one question after another at me about what would happen during the treatment and how long it would take. What she would really have liked was to have a guarantee that it would work. But that is not something that can be predicted. It was difficult for her to cope with the uncertainty. And on top of that she was so bent on getting good results fast and starting her "pregnancy project" that she was constantly asking herself what she was "supposed" to feel during the training, and not what she was really feeling. This made it hard to find the parameters that were right for her, and so I was not surprised that she experienced negative effects. One time she felt dizzy, another time she got a headache. She found this scary and it increased her need to be in control.

In the end I recommended that she continue the treatment with SCP neurofeedback instead. Because in SCP training the client has a task of which they can be consciously aware, the mind has the feeling it can exert an influence on what's happening. I don't know whether she followed my advice. A few years later I saw her at the Christmas Market with two children but they may not have been her own.

Lest I am giving a false impression – it would be wrong to say that one has to "surrender" oneself to ILF neurofeedback. In the vast majority of cases the training does also work with people who don't want to let go of the reins.

5. OBSESSIVE-COMPULSIVE DISORDERS

Obsessive-compulsive behavior can manifest itself in very different ways. Some people can't stop thinking about stressful things. They keep imagining, for example, people they love being killed in an accident or that they themselves offend other people or even do them serious harm. Others have to count everything, keep checking whether the iron is really switched off or they keep washing themselves so frequently and thoroughly that they seriously damage their skin. Sufferers are mostly well aware themselves that their behavior is excessive and pointless, and they try to resist doing it, but usually without success. If they don't manage to carry out a certain desired behavior, they become extremely anxious. This disorder is treated in a similar way to anxiety disorders.

Obsessive-compulsive disorders and neurofeedback

There are many overlaps between anxiety, obsessive-compulsive disorders and eating disorders and from the viewpoint of a neuro-feedback therapist they all have something important in common – they are all rooted in an immense inner tension. In addition to this, in the case of compulsive behaviors the inhibiting effect of the prefrontal cortex is too weak. You will remember that this part of the cerebral cortex is responsible for inhibiting impulsive behaviors (see Part 1, Chapter 1). The patient is not able to interrupt a particular pattern of behavior once it has started. It has not yet been fully explained why this is usually a quite specific, narrowly defined action.

In order to train impulse control in neurofeedback, however, activating tendencies need to be strengthened, and, as you have seen in the case of Justin (see Part 3, Chapter 1), that is not to be recommended in a brain that is already over-excited. For this reason, with obsessive-compulsive disorders, as in ADHD, the therapy begins by calming the nervous system down. Sometimes that is sufficient in itself to prevent the person from carrying out the stereotypical behavior. This was how it was for Nele, whose case I will describe in the following chapter, which deals with eating disorders (see Part 3, Chapter 6).

Too much arousal or too little control?

It is sometimes hard to predict whether a particular behavior is caused by a high level of arousal or by a disinhibition of control. Imagine a champagne bottle with the champagne gushing out of it. That can either happen because the liquid was under very high pressure or because the cork wasn't tightly enough secured. Using a lot of strength to keep the cork in the bottle (suppressing emotions and impulses) is active behavior and associated with a great deal of tension. If the neurofeedback training strengthens our soothing, relaxing and releasing capacities in this situation, this can free up highly emotional behavior – either anger, hysterical laughter or endless sobbing can suddenly pour out.

You may have experienced this when you have had too much to drink or were totally exhausted. Both these scenarios lead to a lowering of inhibitions and can give pointers as to what behavior usually remains "bottled up" – some people become sentimental or tearful, others silly, whiny or aggressive.

For neurofeedback training the key question is how to assess the disinhibition. Sometimes it is positive if suppressed emotions are released, other times one harms oneself. For example, one client's anger boiled over to such an extent that he gave his neighbor a piece of his mind after the session. He felt good about it and said, "Normally I put up with far too much." However, if he had been abusive then his reaction would have had to be judged differently. Crying, laughing and other emotional behaviors can also be counterproductive if they are inappropriately vehement or come at the wrong time.

6. EATING DISORDERS

In order to be able to understand the various pathological disorders of eating behavior it is important to know that although dieting and worrying about their figure and appearance are often the starting point and are what people with these disorders always stress, they are not what drives their behavior. What is characteristic is far more the overpowering desire for control, which is often sparked by a life crisis or mental trauma. However, since most of the circumstances of our lives appear to be largely beyond our control, the desire for control is exercised mainly by subjecting the body to a harsh discipline. This takes the form of an obsession with eating foods that one considers healthy (orthorexia), vomiting after eating (bulimia), fasting or extreme sports training (anorexia). Some people regularly experience a collapse of control, leading to attacks of excessive eating, during which they devour thousands of calories (binge eating, sometimes accompanied by vomiting, sometimes not).

Today we know that people with these disorders also often have brain changes. Thus in binge eaters an area of the cerebral cortex which is responsible for purposeful decisions and impulse control seems to be less active (prefrontal cortex, see Part 1, Chapter 1). Body image disturbance is also typical – anorexic patients have no difficulty recognizing that they are extremely thin when they see themselves in the mirror, but nevertheless they still feel fat. The intellectual recognition that they are underweight remains completely abstract, because what they feel tells them something completely different. The cause could be hormonal disturbances, the "restructuring work" that takes place in the brain during puberty, but it could also be insufficient stimulation of the sensory organs of the skin in all possible ways – bodily contact with other people, digging in the earth with one's bare hands, walking barefoot in a stream, eating with one's fingers, smearing paint and other forms of physical sensuousness.

Various body therapies therefore use methods that exert pressure on the body over an extended period of time – by wrapping the body in towels, for example, or getting the client to wear a made-to-measure wetsuit. The aim is to use this feedback to make the brain aware of the body's true boundaries and overwrite the false inner image, thus correcting the overpowering feeling that often militates against good outcomes in psychotherapy and eating training.

Eating disorders and neurofeedback

The experience gained with neurofeedback treatments is that people suffering from eating disorders have an extremely high arousal level. This is also confirmed by the success of the therapeutic procedure described above – i.e. exerting pressure on the body. This is known to calm the brain. The desire for control leads to a very high level of inner tension and this stress fuels the urge still more. The calming effect of neurofeedback makes it possible to escape this vicious circle. Sometimes it is necessary to combine the treatment with other therapies, but not always. The example of Nele below shows even that it sometimes takes quite a while for the client to learn something from the sessions. The brain simply needs time to internalize new strategies and for these strategies to become a matter of course in how the person behaves in their daily life.

Case example: Anorexia

Delayed success

Nele was in her final year of school when her mother brought her to my office with a diagnosis of "obsessive-compulsive disorder". In fact, the girl's compulsive behavior consisted in her weighing out her meals with great precision and doing a tough weight training session at precisely defined times every day. She found the idea of having a flabby body disgusting – for her everything had to be hard and firm. She had so much tension inside her that she could practically never just sit still, which had become a real problem for her in school and when doing her homework. She was constantly pacing back and forth in their apartment like a tiger – she really did behave like an animal at the zoo in a cage that was far too small for it.

Mother and daughter had a time-consuming journey to get to me and so the sessions were rather less regular than I would have hoped. Despite this we quickly saw some initial improvements – the restless moving around normalized and Nele even started eating with the family again. However, I was skeptical and wondered whether she wasn't doing even more exercise to work off these meals.

After 15 sessions that stretched over a really long period of time because they were at such irregular intervals, the family decided to stop. She was just about to take her school-leaving exams and they just didn't have the time to keep traveling to Stuttgart. I thought it was a pity but that's just how it is sometimes. In my mind I wrote off the treatment as having failed.

But a few months later – a least six months had passed, if not a year – the mother called me to thank me, saying that all the problems had completely disappeared. The pacing around had stopped, there was no mega exercise program, no weighing of meals or any other eating disorders and no other compulsive behavior. Nele was simply a healthy girl again, on the verge of becoming a woman. Her mother was convinced that it was the neurofeedback that had brought about this change, because the family had not tried any other therapy. I was really astonished, because in my view Nele would have needed more sessions to come so far. But at the end it was evidently only the pressure of the exams that had prevented her from putting what she had learned from the neurofeedback into practice in her everyday life.

7. POST-TRAUMATIC STRESS DISORDER (PTSD) / TRAUMATIC STRESS REACTIONS

Post-traumatic stress disorder (PTSD) is an official diagnosis that specifies a strictly defined combination of symptoms which can occur and persist after a person has experienced a traumatic event or series of events. Both persons who have been directly affected and persons who have simply witnessed terrible events can be traumatized.

However, in my view the criteria specified in the PTSD diagnosis fail to capture the broad range of stressors that can provoke traumatic reactions, and they also do not cover all the different manifestations and intensities of these reactions that survivors experience. Most people think that traumatizing experiences have to be extremely threatening events, such as serious accidents, disasters, war and acts of violence. But it has been my experience – which matches that of many trauma experts – that other events such as persistent bullying, poverty, emotional abuse, neglect, severe narcissistic injury and deeply felt losses can also have such a distressing effect on a person that they develop symptoms of trauma.

It is important to understand that traumatization is not something that happens *to* you, but something that happens *inside of* you. It arises when a person's capacity to process a stressful experience psychologically and physically is seriously overwhelmed, leading to various forms of profound emotional and physiological dys-regulation.

A person's memories of a traumatic experience may be fragmentary or, alternatively, sometimes so vivid that they are accompanied by symptoms of physiological hyperarousal or complete shut-down. The person may have haunting nightmares and/or flashbacks in which the boundaries between memory and the current situation and current experience are blurred.

In addition to such reactions, the person is in a constant state of inner alarm that is extremely exhausting and can be the root of various symptoms and disorders. Anxiety disorders, eating disorders and obsessional-compulsive disorders, addictions and borderline syndrome can also often result after experiencing trauma. This state of hyperarousal may also be implicated in many illnesses that are manifested mainly in the body, for example in chronic pain syndromes such as fibromyalgia, autoimmune and skin diseases.

After traumatic experiences people frequently also suffer from feelings of shame and guilt and experience themselves as worthless – it is as if the person was broken inside. Such symptoms often also arise after exposure to a traumatic environment and/or one in which violating actions were perpetrated over a long period and were explicitly directed at the person – in contrast to events such as accidents or natural disasters. Examples are childhood abuse, neglect, domestic violence, slavery and genocidal campaigns.

People who have been traumatized frequently may also experience chronic dissociation. This inner distancing from the world and from the person's own reactions to it is actually a protective mechanism that the psyche employs in order to be able to survive at all. However, if this withdrawal becomes habitual, or has to become so because there is no escape over an extended period, this has serious consequences.

People who react in this way experience an agonizing numbness that stifles all feelings of joy and prevents them from feeling their own emotions and bodily sensations. Not being able to feel yourself properly also makes it very difficult to establish intimacy with other people or even simply to allow it to happen. It is as if one were in a glass bubble or "in the wrong movie" – separated from other people, out of place, and did not belong anywhere. They may find it difficult to imagine a future or be emotionally open and connected to people they are close to.

How severe the consequences of traumatic experiences become depends on what resources are available to help someone cope with them. This is why children can be damaged psychologically by experiences and situations that adults would not consider to be particularly dramatic. What is especially harmful is to be ignored or abandoned by important significant others or to receive little warmth or security from one's parents. In my view there is not sufficient awareness of this when we speak of psychological injury and trauma. Wounds can be caused not only by what one's parents or other significant others do, but also when something essential that we need in order to grow up healthy is lacking. Some experts actually see parental neglect as trauma, since for children it feels, and in fact often is, life-threatening.

Not all traumatized people are aware that they were exposed to overwhelming stress in the past. Some really have no conscious memory of it, while others close their eyes to unpleasant memories. But if we ignore our wounds they may heal over on the surface, but there may still be infected tissue underneath them. When our bodies are injured, the wounded part has to re-form and develop new bone tissue, nails or skin, or scar tissue needs to be able to grow – and psychological wounds need that too. We need to find a way to prevent past events from keeping their hold over us in the present – only then will we be open to new and better experiences. Various psychological, body and art therapies are used to achieve that end, sometimes supported by medication.

Traumatic stress reactions and neurofeedback

Traumatic stress reactions can manifest in many different ways, but nearly all the symptoms are rooted in what I referred to above as a "constant state of inner alarm". The causes of this massive hyperarousal can be treated very effectively with neurofeedback. The brain can learn and is trained to regulate itself better.

Prof. Bessel van der Kolk, a well-known expert on psychological trauma, once said at a conference that neurofeedback is one of the most effective treatments for trauma that he has ever come across. However, this effectiveness is also the reason why therapists need to be trauma-informed. They must create a highly protective setting for the client and be capable of dealing with negative reactions such as anxiety attacks. The client should also be recommended if possible to undergo some other form of trauma-oriented therapy at the same time as the neurofeedback training! This is because improved regulation of the brain is an important prerequisite for sustained change, but it is not sufficient to promote a new, constructive mode of coping with the stressful experiences. This requires additional professional support.

> It is possible to obtain neurofeedback equipment on the internet that can be used at home, however this can be dangerous for very sensitive clients. In people who are less sensitive the difficulty is more that these devices are simply useless. In many cases they do not even record a proper EEG, but rather mainly the activity of the eye and forehead muscles.

Sometimes the opinion is expressed that neurofeedback for trauma patients should only be carried out by their psychotherapists themselves, particularly when childhood development has been disrupted by the traumatization. However, my experience has been that while it is important for the psycho- and neurofeedback therapists to cooperate closely and be in regular contact, it does not need to be one and the same person doing both treatments. The case examples show how this can be done. They were contributed by a trusted colleague who worked in such close cooperation with an experienced psychotherapist that she was even able to treat severely traumatized clients. These cases illustrate once again how it is practically impossible to tell in advance whether a therapy will be successful, and if so, how quickly.

Case example: Post-traumatic stress disorder (1)
From constant vacillation to finding the right way forward

Petra has had various mental health problems all her life. Their roots lie in a childhood that was completely devoid of security. Her mother left her with an aunt when she was still a baby, fetched her back to live with her again later and finally put her in a home. In between she was passed around from one relative to another several times and also abused. Long after she had begun to live alone she was still very wary and only able to relax a little when she was under the influence of drugs and/or alcohol. Although she yearned for stability, she remained restless and would frequently change her job. She had done various therapies but now at 45 her depression was worse than ever and she had the feeling that she was losing control over her life more and more. She was hardly capable of keeping up a front and was afraid that she might soon make mistakes that would cost her her job.

On the advice of her psychotherapist, Petra underwent psychotherapy and also took medication to stabilize her before she came for her first neurofeedback session. Despite this, to begin with the training was difficult. She had many symptoms, which kept changing. This meant that in order to find the right parameters it was necessary for her to have her sessions close together. But she frequently canceled her appointments and it was therefore difficult to adjust the settings to her physical reactions. Her mental state improved, however. She then had a road traffic accident that resulted in a complete setback. The experience itself shocked her. She had to interrupt the neurofeedback treatment and also decided to stop taking her medication while she was in hospital, without consulting her physician. When she came for her next session, mentally she was in the same place she had been in when she first started.

However, what was different from the first attempt was that the therapy had given Petra the feeling for the first time in her life that something had got better. That gave her hope that one day things would finally start improving for her after all. She also surprisingly benefited substantially from a mindfulness course that was offered at the same time. She not only kept coming for the entire eight weeks, but also did the 45-minute daily training. Focusing on her own experience in such a sustained manner for the first time bolstered her motivation enormously. So far she has had a few relapses (rumination, depressed mood, anxiety attacks), but these are happening less and less often. The psychotherapy helps Petra to recognize what triggered these states. It is not yet clear whether she can reach the goal of stopping her medication in a structured way and still remain stable, falling back on therapeutic support only occasionally, as required.

I think it is impressive how much this client was able to achieve in a total of only 30 sessions, despite the fact that her therapy was so irregular and interrupted. The next case example of Samuel shows that the treatment can still be successful even after the most gruesome experiences.

Case example: Post-traumatic stress disorder (2)
Rapidly coming back to life

Samuel had always felt like a stranger in his own family and kept having the impulse to leave. Materially everything was fine, but there was no warmth, as both his mother and his father were undemonstrative and were distant towards him. Both of them came from families who had had to flee at the end of World War 2 and had never really processed those experiences. They never spoke about them. Soon after finishing his training Samuel joined a Christian aid organization and went to work in many different war zones. He now wondered whether the reason for his doing this was because he was working in environments similar to those experienced by his parents. For over 30 years his daily life was determined by war and violence. Again and again he experienced unimaginably brutal scenes. However, for a long time it seemed that he had "packed it all away", as he put it.

Back in Europe, he finally wanted to start leading a quieter life, stop traveling around the world, stay in one place and put down roots. But then he happened to see a house burn down. The frightened screams of a woman and the smoke in the air triggered a whole avalanche of memories that engulfed him as if they were happening in that moment. From that moment on he kept having flashbacks. He was no longer able to cope with hearing voices calling (they didn't even have to be screaming) and would immediately react with intense physical symptoms such as a rapid heartbeat and outbreaks of sweating. He finally started to have panic attacks without any recognizable triggers and found himself in a vortex that kept pulling him further and further down. He was no longer able to sleep and became completely exhausted, depressed and dispirited. What frustrated him most was that he could not work because he felt overwhelmed even by e-mails. He was unable to grasp their content, however often he read them.

Finally Samuel began to do psychotherapy, but it failed to relieve his tremendous tension. He therefore followed his therapist's advice to get neurofeedback treatment. He proved to be one of those people who respond rapidly and intensely to the training. In the first session he therefore initially experienced a few unpleasant reactions such as pressure in his head, dizziness and breathing difficulties. However, once the right settings had been found, not only did these symptoms disappear, but his hopelessness disappeared as well. Amazed, he suddenly realized that he had the feeling that "everything's going to be O.K.".

And it was. After only 20 sessions Samuel had "come back to life" again, as he put it, and was able to stop doing therapy and even to work again. He has not had any flashbacks since.

In view of this client's history it was highly unusual to get such rapid results. This is one more piece of evidence that shows me the enormous potential of ILF neurofeedback. However, it also shows that the method can in no way be considered to be just a "muscle factory for the brain" where the client is simply presented with an equipment pool. The neurofeedback therapist has a powerful tool at their disposal. To conclude the chapter I would therefore like to describe what can happen if the client fails to share painful experiences when their history is taken – either because they don't want to talk about them or because they have completely forgotten them. As the following examples show, that can go well, but sometimes it doesn't.

Case examples: Traumatization

Stressful experiences need to be mentioned!

Britta consulted me because she had frequent headaches. At the initial interview as usual I noted down her symptoms and took her history and also asked specifically about things that stressed her. Somehow I had a feeling ... But she insisted, "No, nothing." But only about two minutes into the first training session she burst out crying. Of course I stopped the treatment immediately and asked her what was happening. She told me she had the feeling that all her stressful experiences were being dissolved and flushed out. She had had no idea how tense she was inside. It turned out that during her childhood she had been exposed to vicious bullying by her classmates for years. While she did experience her crying as sad, she also felt that it was liberating and so she definitely wanted to continue the training. I adjusted the settings so that she would not be so overwhelmed by her feelings.

Tobias, who participated in a beginner's course on neurofeedback, was less lucky. I spoke to him on the morning of the third day because he looked really sick – he was pale and trembling, and he had dark shadows under his eyes. He told me he had not been able to sleep all night because he had been tormented by anxiety and flashbacks. A childhood trauma had surfaced again while he was being treated by another participant as a practice client the day before. The positioning of the electrodes had been unsuitable for someone with his history. Although he had been asked he hadn't said anything because he was embarrassed and thought all that wasn't important anymore. Luckily it was possible to reduce his symptoms considerably after another training session by using the right settings, and by the end of the course he was back where he had been before it started. But this experience had shown him that he needed to take a closer look at his childhood experiences.

8. ADDICTIONS

The development of addiction is usually described as follows: the substances consumed bind to the nerve cell receptors, thus triggering reactions that are similar to the reactions to the body's own neuro-transmitters (see Part 1, Chapter3), but usually appreciably stronger. Over time the neurons become less and less receptive to the signals because the receptors change or become down-regulated so that more and more "dope" is needed to achieve the desired effect. Most drugs act on the brain's reward system, each in its own particular way. The same is also true of compulsive behaviors such as addiction to gaming, sex or shopping, if the person uses it to gain release from a state of unbearable tension or lethargy.

However, this view appears to be wrong – or at least not the whole truth. The British-Swiss celebrity writer and journalist Johann Hari gave a sensational talk entitled "Everything you think you know about addiction is wrong" in which he presented the results of the three years that he had spent looking into this topic in depth. You can watch this video, a TED talk which has had millions of clicks, on www.ted.com. What Hari discovered led him to the conclusion that whether something is addictive or not depends first and foremost on the mental health of the user. He believes that this is one of the reasons why people can take opiates over an extended period of time after serious operations without becoming addicted. "Your granny doesn't come home a junkie after an operation for a hip replacement" he jokes. He argues that if addiction really were only a question of receptors, then it would automatically follow in such cases.

The receptor theory was actually developed on the basis of experi-ments on rats that were given the choice between normal water and water mixed with heroin to drink. The animals almost always preferred the heroin water and got stoned on it until they eventually died. However, Hari quotes the Canadian psychologist Professor Bruce Alexander who looked at the above experiments and realized that the rats had been put in empty cages on their own. He wondered whether the animals' addictive behavior could have simply been due to desperation. So he repeated the experiment, this time putting the rats in an environment that he jokingly called "Rat Park". There were plenty of other rats for company (and also sex), enough room, toys, material to make nests, hiding places, tasty food – and two types of water, one with and one without heroin. The result: on the whole the rats ignored the water with heroin, at most just taking the odd sip of it. There was no addictive drinking and no overdoses.

Alexander's results were later called into question and apparently could not be replicated in other studies. Although I am not able to check the scientific quality of the work of Hari and his critics, I believe his approach is a step in the right direction. Someone who is cared for, who is able to engage in meaningful activities in a congenial environment and leads a life that is integrated in a network of nurturing relationships will not normally develop addictive behavior. But if important basic needs of a person are not met and if they have no security and no support then that will make them susceptible to turning to something else to fill the vacuum.

Addictions and neurofeedback

Experience with neurofeedback supports the above theory, because as a rule therapists use training parameters that are also used in the treatment of early childhood attachment disorders (see appendix). They have a calming effect on inner tension in a way that increases the feeling of security.

But scientific theories of addiction do not in fact play any role in brain training. On the level of the nervous system, addiction is purely and simply an attempt to compensate for a deficit. A person who has an addiction is able to achieve a certain state only, or at least much more easily, through addictive behavior or by consuming the addictive substance. The substances they use give an indication of what it is that is lacking – be it power and focus (amphetamines, ADHD medication, cocaine), harmony and enthusiasm (ecstasy) or calm (alcohol, tranquilizers). Neurofeedback can help the brain to learn how to achieve these states on their own without the need for an addictive substance.

However, as effective as ILF training is in combating drug addiction, if work with addicted persons is to succeed then treatment must take place in an inpatient context with specialized therapists. Patients with addictions need a very clear framework and practitioners need to be really firm and occasionally strict. Neurofeedback is employed very successfully in Norway, for example, but in many other countries it is not yet available. However interest is constantly growing, so I very much hope that this situation will soon change.

9. EPILEPSY

As you know, billions of cells are constantly electrically active in the brain. In an epileptic seizure some or even all of these cells are overexcited – they then all transmit their impulses synchronously. In a seizure that is restricted to a single area (a focal seizure), there are unpleasant sensations or paresthesias and muscle reactions in the areas of the body connected to this part of the brain. However, this focal over-excitation can spread. In generalized epilepsy both sides of the brain are affected, there can be absences (brief episodes of impaired consciousness during which the person does not fall) or a complete loss of control. Muscle spasms can, but may not necessarily, occur in all forms of epilepsy. As a rule the over-excitability of the brain is visible in the EEG, but in about a quarter of patients the recording of the brain waves between attacks is unremarkable.

One special form of epilepsy is what is known as reflex epilepsy. Here the seizures induced by the brain are a response to only a very specific stimulus, which can be highly individual. Some people only have a seizure when listening to a particular piece of music or because of the sensation of a hairbrush on the back of their neck or perhaps when solving problems in geometry. The stimulus gives an indication as to the task of the brain region in question. The trigger is usually a sensitive reaction to visual stimuli (photosensitivity), i.e. contrasting, fast-changing patterns or flashes, for example, as can be found in light shows, films and computer games. Sometimes even the swift typing of text messages is enough to trigger a seizure. People with extreme photosensitivity can protect themselves by wearing glasses with special lenses.

According to the World Health Organization 50 million people world-wide suffer from epilepsy, making this condition one of the most common neurological disorders. Possible causes are acute illness and structural changes brought about by injuries or other harmful factors (drugs for example).

The greater the predisposition to seizures, the more important it is to avoid anything that weakens the body – over-fatigue, extreme physical exertion, alcohol. The illness is usually treated with drugs. Another form of therapy is the ketogenic diet, which is very low in carbohydrates and high in fat. This alters the metabolism so that chemicals called ketones are produced by the fatty acids. These molecules are an excellent source of energy for the brain, which it uses instead of blood glucose (see box for more details). However, it is not yet known why this has an inhibiting effect on the tendency to seizures.

Why the brain loves coconut oil

Coconut oil contains almost exclusively saturated fatty acids that have long been considered unhealthy because of their effect on the cholesterol level. However it has since been shown that this effect stems mainly from an excess of carbohydrates. And this is the line that must be pursued if we are to understand why coconut oil is given a lot of hype for being beneficial in the prevention of Alzheimer's disease and why it is also of interest for the treatment of other brain disorders such as epilepsy.

The brain needs a lot of energy which, in a typical diet, it gets chiefly from glucose, a blood sugar generated from carbohydrates. The processing of fat is too slow for the brain cells, and so an intermediate step is needed. The liver forms substances called ketones from fats, which the brain can then use as "fuel". And this is by no means purely a makeshift solution! It was not until the development of agriculture that this particular supply of energy was side-lined, and, more specifically, only since people have been eating so many easily digestible carbohydrates such as bread, muesli, pasta, rice, cake and also a large amount of sugar. The hormone insulin is almost always used in order to get glucose into the body – and as long as the body has a high insulin level it is hard for ketones to form. In many people this situation becomes worse because the cells increasingly resist the influx of glucose and become less sensitive to insulin. This "insulin resistance" is a preliminary stage of diabetes. It is not noticeable and is not picked up by the conventional blood tests.

But what may seem surprising is that despite there being so much glucose in the body, not enough of it reaches the brain cells. The reason for this is probably that the cells of the vascular system also become insulin-resistant, which means that the blood-brain barrier is harder to cross. This leads to an energy gap that the brain somehow has to close. This deficit is one of the earliest distinctive abnormalities in people who later suffer from Alzheimer's disease. This is possibly also the reason why mental health problems increase the risk of Alzheimer's disease. A brain that is constantly hyper-aroused needs more energy than one that is calm.

If the body has no ketones to offer, the glial cells or glia, which provide the neurons with energy, can also produce some themselves – however to do this they have to break down and "burn" brain matter. In addition to this, a chronic inflammation develops that is probably responsible for the harmful deposits that are most often mentioned with Alzheimer's disease. There are also other factors apart from the lack of energy that can trigger an inflammatory response, such as environmental toxins, for example.

However, when the diet is such that the brain gets ketones from normal metabolic processes, then there are several beneficial effects. Most importantly, the energy gap is closed, the cells obtain a cleaner fuel and this then also has an anti-inflammatory and calming effect on the nerve cells. The ketogenic diet is certainly the most effective method: one eats so few carbohydrates that one's whole metabolism changes. However, for some years there has been criticism of the diet that used to be offered to people with epilepsy. Evidently many of them remain seizure-free with a far less strict diet – in this Modified Atkins Diet (MAD) 10 to 20 grams of carbohydrate are permitted per day and as much protein as one likes. This is important for children, especially, as they need these nutrients for growth.

But there is also a way of providing the brain with ketones that requires less discipline – coconut oil. This contains an unusually large amount of medium-chain fatty acids (MCTs or medium-chain triglycerides) that are converted to ketones in the liver, regardless of how many carbohydrates are included in the diet. Currently more and more researchers are beginning to investigate the effect of coconut oil on Alzheimer's disease, both as a preventive measure and on those who already have initial symptoms. Thus far research has consisted mainly of single-case studies, but these have produced hopeful results. As long as not too much brain tissue has been destroyed, patients can often really improve their situation.

According to what we know so far, anyone who is already aware of a decline in their brain function should take a dessert spoon of cold-pressed virgin coconut oil at regular intervals five times a day, two are enough as a preventive measure. If you choose a really high quality oil, you can hardly go wrong, because when it cools, the creamy white fat is very digestible and tastes wonderful. It can be used for frying vegetables, adding to soups, and pepping up muesli and smoothies.

As a next step it would be interesting to look at whether people with other brain function disorders might also be able to benefit from coconut oil, and see whether neurofeedback training would be even more effective if the brain were to get this high quality fuel.

Epilepsy and neurofeedback

As mentioned in Part 2, above, the treatment of epilepsy with frequency band training marked the birth of neurofeedback therapy, and this has continued to be used with great success for the last 40 years. Today SCP training is also often employed. Whereas in most disorders the training consists of working intensively on both the up- and down-regulation of excitability, with epilepsy the important thing is to reduce it. In particular, a study group run by the neurologists Professor Niels

Birbaumer and Ute Strehl at Tübingen University in Germany has demonstrated in many studies that patients treated by neurofeedback are able to reduce the number of seizures they have – and sometimes have no more seizures at all. It has now also been shown that these effects of the therapy are sustained, even lasting as long as ten years.

> Many epilepsy sufferers complain that over time their mental capacities are reduced by the seizures. A second Tübingen study monitored IQ levels after SCP training and found that it raises the IQ level again.

Fewer studies have been conducted on ILF training, but there are a number of single case studies with rigorous designs. The results of these confirm my own experience and that of many colleagues that ILF feedback produces very good results in epilepsy. One example of this is Marco.

Case example: Epilepsy
Hope for Marco

Ten year old Marco was suffering from serious epilepsy and having violent seizures several times a week. Strong medication had no effect at all. When Marco consulted me there was some discussion as to whether to increase the dosage even more, but the drugs were really knocking him out already. Sedating him even more with drugs would not only have had a serious effect on his quality of life, but would also have made it impossible for him to continue going to school. He was already suffering from memory problems that impaired his ability to learn. In their search for alternative solutions the parents discovered neurofeedback.

Marco looked forward to the training. He came twice a week and would take the music that he listened to during the sessions home with him. This supported him in his daily life at home. After just four sessions he had no more grand mal seizures. However, it took longer to stabilize his brain even further. It wasn't until he had done 40 sessions (i.e. about six months later) that there was no more talk of increasing the medication. In fact the opposite was the case – his doctors were considering reducing it. Marco continued with the training, although less frequently, and hoped that one day he might possibly be able to lead a life free of seizures without having to take any pills at all.

However, there are a few exceptions. In the worst case scenario the training can even trigger a seizure before the therapist has found the right individual settings for the client. For this reason it is necessary to be extremely cautious. If there is an interval of several weeks between seizures the therapist has to rely on there being symptoms also during this interval – otherwise it is very hard to check the changes that have been triggered by the training. Some clients do not have symptoms during this time or are not able to describe their symptoms very well – then I have to depend on my experience alone and I'm more or less working in the dark. So when I have clients who are really afraid of a seizure, I prefer to send them to SCP training.

10. MIGRAINE

It is an error to believe that it is mainly women who suffer from migraine. According to studies conducted by the German Migraine and Headache Society[4], 40 per cent of the roughly 8 million people who suffer from migraine in Germany are men. Sometimes the severity of the illness is played down and every headache is referred to as migraine, just as people fail to differentiate between real flu and a common cold. In fact, migraine can rob sufferers of a large part of their life – and also of the joy of life, which can be substantially diminished not only by the pain itself, but also by worrying about the next attack.

Once a migraine has begun, usually the only thing that helps is undisturbed rest and waiting for it to pass in a room that is as quiet as possible, fighting against the nausea and somehow enduring with the pulsating headache. Anything more than that is simply too much, and that sometimes goes on for hours on end, sometimes even for days on end. This is followed by a phase of severe exhaustion, which can also last a whole day.

There are several theories as to how migraine develops. They are not necessarily mutually exclusive, but seem to mesh with each other. The pain evidently arises through the blood vessels over-expanding in the brain. At the same time the tissue becomes puffed up, a process in which inflammatory factors are also involved. This explains the typical pulsating character of the pain, but not the neurological symptoms. Some migraine sufferers have visual, sensory or speech disturbances just before an attack begins, which are called an aura. We now know that these phenomena develop because the cells in the affected areas

---

4   **Ger.** Deutsche Migräne- und Kopfschmerzgesellschaft

of the cerebral cortex briefly become over-excited, and then "switch off" for a while. Whether and how these phenomena are involved in the development of the pain that follows is not clear.

A central role is played in the pain process by the trigeminus nerve which is a cranial nerve and, as its name says, has three branches that radiate to the front of the head. This is evidently where most migraine attacks start. However, why the trigeminus nerve is irritated is still somewhat of a mystery. There are indications that inflammation and an imbalance in the neurotransmitters could be involved. Another possible factor is mechanical overload arising from the person grinding their teeth at night, or bruxism. This is also a sign that they are "chewing their way through" a stressful situation.

This also applies to changes in sleep rhythm, which are one of the major triggers of attacks. They may be a trigger in their own right, or they may be a sign that the person is currently under too much pressure. Other triggers are certain foods, fluctuations in hormone levels, changes in air pressure, glaring light, flashes or flickering images, as can arise when there are when moving in and out of the sun and shade.

Triptans are the drugs most widely used in the treatment of migraine. They are only effective in the treatment of migraine symptoms, and then only if they are taken at an early stage in the course of an attack. If a person has more than three migraines a month, the attacks last for longer than 48 hours or cannot be controlled with painkillers, triptans can be taken prophylactically, either alone or in combination with other medications. Migraine is also treated with a new class of medication called CGRP inhibitors and various naturopathic methods such as homeopathy, acupuncture and osteopathy.

Migraine and neurofeedback

Research has shown that migraine patients always react hypersensitively to stimuli, and not only during an attack. Their brains also do not adapt to stimuli that recur. They are not "filtered out", but raise the excitability of the brain more and more, to the point where an attack is triggered. As with epilepsy, the area under the top of the arousal-performance curve (where migraine patients feel good is very narrow.

While it has now been ruled out that there is such a thing as a "migraine personality", there are in fact migraine sufferers who do share some commonalities. They are often achievement-oriented and highly motivated people who push themselves to the limit. They often have jobs that involve a lot of thinking and little exercise: a lot of work for the head and not much for the body. But is a migraine attack really something like an emergency switch, because it forces the sufferer to avoid all stimuli if they can? I have my doubts, because many migraine sufferers have an attack at the very moment they want to switch from activity to relaxation. For example, one of my clients would always get a migraine when he stepped into a hot bath. It could be that those people keep pushing themselves as long as they can because they are unconsciously aware that letting go could trigger an attack.

Luckily it is not necessary to know the answer to the question as to what comes first in order to be able to help migraine patients. ILF training teaches them to lower the excitability of their brain and to switch more easily between active and relaxing states. The sentinel net-work is also strengthened so that it becomes more efficient at filtering out unimportant stimuli.

If the SCP method is employed it can also be combined with biofeedback. With this procedure the patient learns to reduce the dilatation of the blood vessels in the brain and can slow down an incipient attack or even stop it.

Because migraine patients react extremely sensitively, therapists should be very cautious when adjusting the settings and not try too much at once. For clients it is important to know that the treatment does not cause the brain to lose its vulnerability completely – it is only that its "buffer" becomes bigger, as shown by the case of Sabine, below.

Case example: Migraine
More breathing space for Sabine

Sabine was 36 years old and was well aware of what her migraine triggers were: stress, an irregular sleep-wake rhythm, her premenstrual hormonal changes and red wine. It is easy not to drink something that doesn't agree with you, but the other triggers are more difficult to avoid. Sabine therefore decided to try neurofeedback and was largely free of migraines after only ten sessions. Euphorically she said, "Migraines? I don't have them any more!"

However, that wasn't quite the case, as she later discovered. Now she puts it this way: "Before, a single trigger was enough for me to get a migraine. Today I only get one if three triggers come at once." In other words, the therapy has expanded her "breathing space", but she still has to take care of herself in order not to bring on an attack.

11. CHRONIC PAIN

Many people think of pain as being something objective – the more serious the cause, the more it hurts. In actual fact, how much pain we feel depends on many factors, our frame of mind being particularly important. Someone who is undergoing a lot of stress, is feeling lonely or sad or even depressed, will be more sensitive to unpleasant irritations than someone who is in really good shape. The same applies to people who are anxiously keeping every little ache and pain under observation. Disturbed sleep also greatly increases pain. Pain specialists believe the cause lies in the brain. In people who don't get a relaxing night's sleep the brain evidently reacts in a more sensitive way to irritations.

> According to the International Association for the Study of Pain, using data from the World Health Survey 2002 –200, the overall prevalence of pain across countries was estimated to be 27.5%, with significant variation across countries (ranging from 9.9% to 50.3%).

In all of these circumstances there is also an increased risk that pain will become chronic or even become an illness in its own right, because even harmless stimuli are perceived as being painful or because the pain from an injury or illness persist long after the cause has disappeared. In such cases a "pain memory" has formed. To stop this happening, specialists stress the importance of treating pain after operations, for example.

A wide variety of procedures, in both conventional and complementary medicine, are used to treat chronic pain, ranging from acupuncture and arthroscopy to suppositories and Zen meditation. It is increasingly becoming accepted that patients benefit most from "multimodal therapy", which accords equal importance to mental and the physical health. This is particularly the true for "functional" pain that is caused not by tissue damage but by tense or cramped muscles.

Chronic pain and neurofeedback

Neurofeedback can be very successful in alleviating the tension that causes or intensifies pain. In fact, sometimes neurofeedback is all that is needed, as proved to be the case with Jürgen, see below. However, no amount of brain training will help in the case of persistently poor posture – the muscles (also) need to be exercised and strengthened. For this reason neurofeedback is most effective if it is used in conjunction with physiotherapy. We particularly like to advise patients to book appointments for massage, chiropractic treatment or training of the specific muscles involved straight after the neurofeedback session.

Case example: Chronic pain (1)
Jürgen becomes pain-free

Jürgen had had "back problems" ever since he started work. He knew it was "just" tension, but sometimes it made his life hell. He needed a course of heat treatment and massage at least twice a year to be able to "function again", as he put it. But what was causing the pain remained a mystery to him as he was by no means a couch potato.

A friend told him about neurofeedback and Jürgen came to my clinic to in search of a different solution to his muscular tension. After a few sessions he realized what was wrong. He had always got worked up over everything, would hit the roof over the smallest thing and was hardly ever prepared to just let things go. He would always get the tension when he went to a restaurant or on holiday and practically every time he had any dealings with officials. Of course it was the "chicken or the egg" problem – was he tense because he was constantly getting angry or did he erupt straight away because of the tension inside him? Fortunately neurofeedback doesn't have to answer such questions in order to produce results. "It's as if a switch has flipped", Jürgen said after six sessions and appeared really relaxed. His back pain gradually eased and we were able to end the treatment after 20 sessions.

It later emerged that the "switch" really was the right one for Jürgen's back pain. Because when I ran into him three years later he told me that he no longer needed any physiotherapy to remain pain-free. Then he hesitated and laughed, "That did the trick then, no more physical problems."

Even when a "pain memory" has formed, neurofeedback can still help with the unlearning of this now meaningless reaction. However, if even intensive ILF Training has no effect on chronic pain at all, then we need to be suspicious. As proved to be the case with my client Heide (see below), the root of the problem is usually in fact structural damage.

Case example: Chronic pain (2)
Neurofeedback is not magic

Heide was suffering from intense pain in the lumbar region and could hardly stand upright. Sleep was also – completely out of the question. She had consulted numerous doctors but none of them had been able to find what was causing the pain. They all thought that it was tension. However, neither muscle relaxing injections nor physiotherapy or acupuncture did any good at all. She could only struggle up the steps to my clinic one step at a time, it was sheer agony for her.

And there was no change at all even after several neurofeedback sessions. She was not sleeping any better either. Following my advice Heide got an appointment for an examination at a specialist clinic with the most modern X-ray techniques, and lo and behold – there was a slipped disc which was pressing so hard on the nerve that she had to have surgery. This really did result in the longed-for relief and after undergoing rehabilitation Heide was functioning almost as well as before.

This shows that the cause of the pain has to be the point of departure in neurofeedback. Otherwise brain training can have little effect – and in extreme cases no effect at all.

12. STRESS

Are you surprised that we haven't got to stress before, and now we're right at the end, after eleven chapters dealing with serious disturbances of brain function that can have a huge effect on people's lives and also on those of their relatives? Don't most people suffer from stress?

Of course they do! One out of every two people, to be precise. In all the studies on stress about half of those asked say they feel permanently stressed. Of course we can assume that some people are just saying that mainly because it's the thing to have a hectic life style. But it doesn't alter the fact that the number of people who feel they're chasing their own tail is huge.

If you've got up to here in this book you will have realized that it does the brain no good at all to overstimulate it and that this can lead to all manner of mental and physical symptoms.

In this world where everything is controlled by technology we keep forgetting that we human beings are not machines. If we are really going to function well we need time to warm up, to ease off gently, and we need transitions and downtime. It is precisely these "unproductive" moments that all those people who are obsessed with time management would really like to get rid of. But it is a mistake to believe that procedures that are as tightly run as possible are the most efficient! And yet a lot of people pursue are fixated on this idea, even in those areas of their everyday lives where they make their own decisions, and are then surprised that they never get what they most long for – time affluence. Having the leisure to do whatever they happen feel like, whether it's a job that has to be done or sitting down with a good book.

The more tightly regimented our working days are, the less likely it is that we will be able to stop the "constant running around" when it's time to go home. Many of us find it literally impossible to switch off, above all because of modern media. The overburdening of our nervous systems caused by the constant inflow of information is now so widespread that experts have a special name for it – "digital burnout" (see box).

Digital Burnout – when it's impossible to switch off

Modern media are having an extremely fragmenting effect on many people's everyday lives. According to a comprehensive study conducted by the University of Bonn in Germany, on average people use their smartphones 53 times a day – 90% of the time for text messages, games, and catching up with the news and social media (this doesn't include listening to music). According to Alexander Markowetz, who is in charge of the study, on top of this people check their phones 35 times a day without doing anything. The average person uses their phone for online communication for a total of three to four hours a day. The more time they spend doing this, the more signs of addictive behavior become evident. The first thing they do in the morning is check their messages, they are constantly available, extremely afraid of missing something and become agitated if there happens to be no signal. Smartphones can in fact have the same effect on the brain as gambling, because every click promises a surprise.

But even in cases where addictive behavior is not, or not yet, an issue it is impossible to relax and concentrate on your work when something is constantly ringing, buzzing or popping up. Studies on flow, that wonderful state of being completely immersed in what you are doing, have shown that it takes up to 15 minutes to be able to fully immerse yourself in a task again after an interruption. If you keep getting disturbed before that point, you will never experience the state of flow. Also, there will always be a gradual increase in internal tension if the brain is constantly being bombarded with input.

Being constantly available becomes stressful if you are also faced with work messages outside working hours. For many people the digital freedom that enables us to work anywhere or at any time has become a curse, since it now means being permanently digitally available. We can, quite literally, never switch off, and this may, under certain circumstances, cause such psychological stress that we end up with "digital burnout". More and more firms are also beginning to recognize the problem. This is why some of them turn their email servers off in the evening, for example. Some also employ coaches who specialize in teaching firms and their employees healthier online habits. However, some people have so much inner tension that coaching alone is no longer any use. In such cases neurofeedback can, among other things, help the brain to get back into a more relaxed state.

There are also things you can do yourself. You can switch off your phone more often. You can use an app such as "Offtime" that blocks calls and notifications but allows you to create specific contact exceptions so that important callers can still get through. Deactivate all the signals that show that emails are coming in and deal with these only a few times a day. Reduce the flood of mobile data – no emails on your phone, no push notifications. Turn all your devices off completely two hours before you go to bed, not just because of all the messages coming in, but because the blue light that the screen emits can disturb your sleep.

But even if you are not an online addict and you don't overload your evenings and weekends with activities, the fact is that nobody automatically relaxes just because work is over for the day or it's Sunday or holidays are coming up. The faster you're moving, the longer it takes to brake! Occasional periods of "downtime" can be a good thing, but basically this only serves to prepare you to be part of the machinery again. And to use the driving metaphor again, do you think your engine would recover if you drove it for a short way at walking pace, if the rest of the time you were always driving like a racing driver? Exactly! And it's the same with all the disorders that we've looked at in the previous chapters. Brains work best at optimal revs – sometimes a bit faster or slower, but never at revs that are too high or too low.

Stress and neurofeedback

You can, of course, use neurofeedback to help you get into this rev range more easily, even if you don't have a serious diagnosis. However, if you see the training simply as a way of getting that hamster wheel turning a bit faster, I will have to disappoint you. That would be going back to the idea that the brain is a computer. And neurofeedback therapy is not an update for your hard drive that will enable you to push yourself even harder. Although the sessions can feel restful, the effect will not be sustained if nothing else changes in your life. We can see this from the example of disturbed sleep. Neurofeedback training can help you fall asleep more quickly and wake up feeling more refreshed, but that's no use at all if you don't get yourself to bed, but end up working late into the night.

It is rare that people come to me wanting me to give their brains a boost so that they can push themselves even harder at work. Most want to regain the ability to enjoy their work again. We see this in the example of Heike, who felt that she was heading for a burnout.

Case example: Stress
Five minutes to burnout – just in time

Heike came to my office because she had read an article about burnout that really shook her. She hadn't reached that stage yet, she said, but she was already aware of a few warning signs, the most prominent being difficulty sleeping. This 37 year old woman was finding it hard to get to sleep, had night sweats, was tortured by dreams about work and often would often wake up in the early hours. She felt as if she was being dragged into a whirlpool of exhaustion which was making her work feel unbearably demanding and hard and was draining all the pleasure/any pleasure she had in it. The reason for this was less the workload as such but rather the fact that she couldn't stop thinking about work when she came home at the end of the day. So far she had tried to "invest a lot of effort in relaxing" (her choice of words says it all!) by doing exercise, autogenic training and getting spa treatments. Sometimes these things helped, but there were other evenings when she was jogging or in a meditation class or the sauna and her head would just carry on working and she couldn't stop worrying.

It wasn't until she did neurofeedback that she realized that the real solutions are to be found elsewhere. The training made her brain more able to protect her from all the stimuli that were raining down on her and just engage in things that seemed sensible at the time. This also meant actively setting limits, such as closing her office door, sometimes making herself unavailable, not opening every email straight away or not instantly reacting to every small thing. She learned to tell her colleagues "I'll just finish this and then I'll come and see you". All of these things gave her the feeling of being able to decide important aspects of her work herself, of not being so driven any more. And in the end she gradually took pleasure in her work again.

Because Heike did something about it in time, her symptoms quickly improved. She still had resources inside her that she only had to reactivate, unlike clients who don't start the training until they've already had a breakdown. Before long we were able to increase the time gaps between appointments and we ended the treatment completely after six months.

The reason why neurofeedback was such a great help to Heike was because she brought on most of her problems herself with all her ruminating, which ate into her energy. The training helped her to more easily get into states of relaxation, without which changes would not be possible at all. If you are in a state of hyperarousal all you do is stare problems in the face – but solutions that can really work are mostly just out of view.

However, many people are afraid of taking a closer look at things. They also avoid taking proper moments of relaxation because they instinctively feel that lurking somewhere in their inner junk room there is the deep pain of missed opportunities and unfulfilled desires. If you were really just to take a moment to pause, you might possibly run the risk of realizing that you are wearing yourself out in a job that doesn't suit you at all – and what then? I can only encourage you to take the risk, because you have everything to gain. You can't stop and turn back in life, but you can always correct the course you are on, as we see in the example of Linda.

Case example: Life crisis
There's always something you can do

Linda came to see me when she was in her early sixties. She was in a crisis because a serious life-changing event had suddenly made her question everything. To start with the neurofeedback training slowed down all the thoughts going round in her head and calmed the system. After a few sessions she came to realize that at certain times in her life she really had "taken a wrong turning". But instead of just blindly carrying on and stubbornly ignoring what she was doing, she consciously said goodbye to all that might have been. "There are some things I wish I'd done differently", she said, giving herself permission to be sad about it. And then she let it go and turned her gaze towards the future again. Instead of allowing herself to be get depressed about it she focused anew on all the things that were still possible. So she moved to a new department at work, for example, and reduced her hours. And suddenly she had lots of time to paint and do all those other things that she'd never dared do or given herself permission to do in the past.

Even when your own life feels completely messed up, it's rarely necessary to give everything up in order to find peace and happiness. Get some help! There are coaches, therapists, courses, books, DVDs and countless numbers of inspiring talks to listen to on the internet. It has never been so easy to find someone to show you paths you might take towards leading a more fulfilled life. But only you can actually start out on these paths, not even neurofeedback treatment can do that for you.

MORE CHILL-OUT TIME FOR THE BRAIN!

I am sure that by now you've grasped my passion for neurofeedback. In the hands of a responsible therapist it is an immensely effective tool for stimulating the brain's capacity to develop. However, it's not the only one as we now know – yoga, meditation and mindfulness practice have similar effects. The difference is that neurofeedback gives people a stronger "prod in the back" and is at the same time something that is easier to access. You just have to do a bit of watching or playing! People can manage that even if their nervous system is so out of balance that they aren't able to benefit from regular meditation, for example.

However, the greater your own resources, the greater your ability to strengthen your brain yourself and keep it capable of developing. What is important here is that special state in which the brain is awake but does not have to perform any tasks. This is the state we call chilling out. A short walk in the woods or listening to some lovely music can put the brain into this mode, as can painting, for example, when we become completely oblivious of our surroundings, or just gazing into space. Many people have completely forgotten what it is to be chilled out, and even when they are having the most wonderful massage, they are still mentally ticking off what's to be done on their to-do-list. But don't let this put you off. People who are moving at a high speed simply need a longer time to brake before they arrive. The more often and the more thoroughly you practice, the easier it is for your brain to be able to switch to "standby mode" and back again. I am convinced that I would have far fewer patients if refreshing the brain for 30 –50 minutes every day was as natural as cleaning one's teeth or having a shower.

So give your brain the chance to experience the conditions it needs to be able to develop. It needs rest just as much as it needs stimulation–breaks, sleep, fresh air and exercise. Clear your diary of all the "Must do's and make space for things that really bring you pleasure. Of course, being able to work in a focused way is good, but alongside that there should also be plenty of time to dawdle, dream and purely and simply enjoy. Only if you can offer the "dough" between your ears all of that, can it rise. And that is when all the kneading really pays off.

Meike Wiedemann

APPENDIX

Below you will find a list of symptoms and complaints that can be positively influenced by neurofeedback and especially by ILF training. The list is impressively long, mainly because the dysregulation of the brain of course also has an effect on the autonomic nervous system, leading to a wide variety of bodily symptoms. However, as wide-ranging as the possibilities of neurofeedback are, you should always make an appointment with your doctor for a check-up before trying it.

Abdominal cramps / pain
See Pain / Hormonal disturbances / Digestive problems

ADD/ADHD
See detailed description in Part 3, Chapter 1

Addictive and substance use disorders
See detailed description in Part 3, Chapter 8

Aggression
Anger that is boiling over responds very well to neurofeedback and in many disorders it is one of the first symptoms to disappear.

Alzheimer's disease
Neurofeedback training can have positive effects in cases of de-generative brain diseases such as Alzheimer's disease, but it is not clear to what extent. Some therapists report that the training makes their dementia patients more alert and receptive. Recent studies in mice have shown that gamma frequencies may slow down the development of harmful plaques in the brain. However, the training should begin as

soon as possible after the initial signs of dementia become evident with a view to keeping going with it.

See also Brain damage.

Anorexia nervosa
See Eating disorders.

Anxiety disorders
See detailed description in Part 3, Chapter 4

Asperger's syndrome
See Autism

Asthma
See Breathing difficulties

Attachment disorders
Children need at least one reliable relationship in order to be able to develop well mentally. If a person is unable to experience such an attachment relationship or had one that was disrupted in sensitive phases (e.g. if their mother was sick) this is often later evidenced in a lack of trust on the deepest level. As a result the person is not able to experience the associated open, relaxed state, or only rarely. Neurofeedback can help the brain to access such states and thus enable it to have new experiences. Psychotherapy can then be much more effective.

However, if a person has simply been hurt in a relationship with a partner and subsequently shies away from starting a new relationship, that is not as a rule an indication for neurofeedback.

Attention deficit (hyperactivity) disorder
See AD(H)D

Autism spectrum disorders

See detailed description in Part 3, Chapter 2

Bedwetting

See Incontinence

Binge eating

See Eating disorders

Bipolar disorders

See detailed description in Part 3, Chapter 3

Blanking out

See Fainting fits and Exam / Test anxiety

Blood pressure

See Stress

Borderline disorder

The word borderline is used to mean that the disorder is somewhere in the intermediate zone between psychosis and neurosis. Thus a person suffering from schizophrenia (psychosis), for example, is not able to tell whether voices that they hear are in their head or come from outside. In contrast, patients with borderline disorder know very well which perceptions are real and which are not. What distinguishes them from persons with neurotic problems are mainly their emotional outbursts, which can be triggered by very small things. For them, anger, despair, mistrust and anxiety, also passion and love are boundless. Their needs pull them in two extreme directions at once and plunge them into an extreme inner tension in which they are hardly able to feel or sense themselves at all anymore. Some of them self-harm, which gives them some relief.

Since the high level of arousal is in the foreground in this disorder it is highly accessible to neurofeedback treatment. However, the therapist needs to be very familiar with the disorder. In severe cases the treatment is best carried out in an inpatient context.

Brain damage

When nerve connections are damaged – irrespective of whether the cause was a stroke, poisoning, an infection, an accident or simply infirmity due to old age – the cells affected do not necessarily stop conducting electric impulses. Instead they may transmit signals that are irregular, too strong or unsuitable in some other way and thus disrupt whole networks. The brain then has difficulty in filtering meaningful signals out of this "noise", particularly in challenging situations. Neurofeedback can help to calm down the "noisy" brain and to resynchronize the networks that have become muddled. The person is then able to relearn the skills that they have lost.

Breathing difficulties

Since in many cases breathing problems are caused by stress, or at least aggravated by it, these can be alleviated by neurofeedback.

Bruxism

See Teeth grinding

Bulimia

See Eating disorders

Burnout

See detailed description in Part 3, Chapter 3

Cardiovascular disorders

See Stress

Constipation

Where constipation is a symptom of hyperarousal it can often be permanently cured with the help of neurofeedback.
See also Digestive problems

Dementia

See Alzheimer's disease / Brain damage

Depression

See detailed description in Part 3, Chapter 3

Diarrhea

If the diarrhea is a symptom of a dysregulation of the arousal level or has psychosomatic roots it often responds well to neurofeedback. See also Digestive problems.

Difficulty concentrating

See Stress / AD(H)D

Digestive problems

If you are constantly bothered by stomach cramps, diarrhea and constipation, the underlying reason is often a food intolerance, e.g. a sensitivity to the wheat protein gluten, lactose (milk sugar), fructose (fruit sugar), the artificial sweetener sorbitol or the protein histamine. In contrast to the case with true allergies, it often requires real detective work to find the cause. If you have such a sensitivity, neurofeedback is usually unsuccessful. For example, if there is no change in migraine after a few sessions you should get tested for histamine intolerance.

However, digestive problems can also occur when the activity of the stomach is disturbed. It doesn't move in the way it should to be able to process food as needed. As a consequence, too little of the enzymes required for digestion is secreted or this doesn't happen when it should. This is usually due to too much stress and rushing around and it can therefore help if you simply make sure that you have more time and peace and quiet at mealtimes. However, if your inner tension is so high that this alone fails to lead to much of an improvement, neurofeedback can help.

See also Stress.

Disturbances of vision
Only when the cause is in the brain can neurofeedback lead to an improvement, and not when the damage is structural.

Dizziness / vertigo
Since dizziness can be a symptom of very many illnesses it is important to identify the possible causes first. If no cause is found then neurofeedback therapy can be tried. It can be successful in those types of dizziness that are related to muscular tension or those that come on suddenly, as attacks.

See also Menière's disease

Eating disorders
See detailed description in Part 3, Chapter 6

Eczema
See Skin problems

Epilepsy
See detailed description in Part 3, Chapter 9

Exam / Test anxiety

For some people the nervousness that is quite normal before taking an exam or test, giving a lecture or appearing on stage is so great that they suffer from severe physical problems such as stomach ache, vomiting, diarrhea or palpitations. They underperform badly, their minds go blank or they even fail completely. Neurofeedback helps greatly with such severe feelings of stress (see also Stress). It also helps with a different phenomenon that professional musicians sometimes complain of – they are technically highly proficient and also capable of performing perfectly at a moment's notice, but they don't enjoy it. They "produce" music and sometimes feel like robots. Neurofeedback can help them to practice balancing control and relaxation and in turn to play their instrument (again) and not to use it as a piece of equipment.

Fainting fits

Many illnesses can be responsible for a tendency to faint and it is important to explore these as possible reasons first. If the cause cannot be found, neurofeedback therapy could be tried because, it is precisely when there is a sudden onset that some instability of the brain may be involved.

Fibromyalgia

See Pain

Headaches

See Tension headaches / Migraine

Heart /circulation Problems

See Stress

Hormonal disturbances

Since the regulation of hormone secretion is closely linked to the nervous system, neurofeedback can often help to re-establish a more healthy balance. However, the thyroid gland needs to be considered separately because it is more like a conductor than a member of the orchestra, and has a strong effect on the level of arousal. Thus, the dosage of medications for disorders of hormone function should be well adjusted before any neurofeedback treatment.

Hyperactivity

See AD(H)D

Hyperhidrosis

See Sweating

Incontinence

If a person is unable to control their bladder or their bowel movements or cannot prevent themselves from breaking wind, biofeedback is the treatment of choice, rather than neurofeedback. An exception is bedwetting. Incontinence is a frequent symptom in children who present with other diagnoses and usually disappears relatively fast.

Irritable bowel syndrome (IBS)

If the symptoms have a psychosomatic background they respond well to neurofeedback.
See also Digestive problems.

Itching (pruritus)

Studies show that many people suffer from chronic itching (lasting for more than six weeks) without consulting a doctor. However, this excruciating symptom can be an indication of a number of disorders, such as diabetes, kidney and liver disease and also disorders of hematopoiesis (defective blood formation). Surprisingly often, however, the cause is simply lactose intolerance or an intolerance of the artificial sweetener sorbitol. Patients who have pruritus must seek expert medical help to determine the cause of the problem. In some cities and regions there are specialized clinics. It is also recommended to get expert help even if the cause for the itching is known, as chronic itching can create a memory, in the same way that pain can. If that happens, despite the fact that the original cause has long been dealt with, the itching persists. In such a case neurofeedback can help the brain to reorganize itself and "unlearn" the itching. Similarly, neurodermatitis, which is closely connected to the nervous system, responds well to training.

Lower abdominal pain
See Pain / Hormonal disturbances / Digestive problems

Menière's disease
In this condition a disturbance of pressure in the inner ear leads to sometimes overwhelming attacks of vertigo that can result in complete collapse. The fact that attacks come on suddenly indicates that there may be some instability in the brain that plays a part. In this case neurofeedback can support the treatment.

Menopausal discomfort
See Hormonal disturbances

Migraine
See detailed description in Part 3, Chapter 10

Muscle cramps and tension
See Pain / Stress

Neurodermatitis
See Skin problems

Obsessive-compulsive behaviors
See detailed description in Part 3, Chapter 5.

Orthorexia nervosa
See Eating disorders

Pain
See detailed description in Part 3, Chapter 11

Parkinson's disease
In this disease, cells that produce the neurotransmitter dopamine die. As a result people suffering from it have a strong tremor and at the same time they have difficulty in initiating goal-directed movements. Their facial expressions also become increasingly rigid. Although neuro-feedback cannot change the cause, it still often has a strong positive effect on the typical symptoms.

Phobias
See Anxiety disorders

Post-traumatic stress disorder (PTSD) / Traumatic stress reactions
See detailed description in Part 3, Chapter 7

Premenstrual syndrome
See Hormonal disturbances/Pain

Pruritus
See Itching

Sensory disorders

When the cause of abnormal sensations, such as changes in the sense of smell or taste, is to be found in the brain, neurofeedback can lead to an improvement, but not if the problem is due to structural damage.

Skin problems

Since in many cases skin problems are caused, or at least aggravated, by stress, neurofeedback has a positive effect on them.

Sleep disturbances

The first signs of success of neurofeedback training are often that client's sleep greatly improves. Even persistent cases of disturbed sleep respond well to therapy. Sometimes it helps to use frequency band training as well (Alpha synchrony or Alpha/Theta), to learn to let go and drift into the relaxed in-between state before dropping off to sleep.

Sports performance

Neurofeedback can help ambitious sportsmen and women attain various different states more directly. It is not simply a question of peak performance levels, but also of being able to recover effectively. You can really only recuperate if you manage to cast aside the exertion of an intensive training session or a contest. Many sportsmen and women only learn how to get charged up – but in order to stay fit and competitive you always have to be able to come down again.

Stage fright

See Exam / Test anxiety

Stress

See detailed description in Part 3, Chapter 12

Stroke

See Brain damage

Stuttering

As we now know the causes of these speech difficulties lie in the brain. Disturbances of metabolism have been found in the various different speech centers of the cortex and excessive activity of the neurotransmitter dopamine is assumed to be the cause. In many cases the problem disappears with time: up to 60 to 80 per cent of children who stutter no longer stutter by the time they reach adulthood. Neurofeedback can help to accelerate this process and thus save the children much distress. The training is particularly effective when it is combined with speech therapy.

Sweating

Excessive sweating (hyperhidrosis) can be restricted to individual parts of the body or it can be "general". The reason for breaking out into a complete sweat is usually hormonal disturbances, as can happen during the menopause for example. The reason for more localized sweating, on the other hand, is to be found in the brain, or more precisely in the hypothalamus giving the wrong signals to the sweat glands. In some people it is their hands and feet that sweat (in rare cases only one of the two), in others the armpits or the head or a combination of both. Whereas in healthy people perspiration builds up in a linear way – the more they exercise or become excited, the more they sweat – in hyperhidrosis the curve grows exponentially. In other words, the body parts affected break out into an extreme sweat at the slightest provocation.

There is a therapy called iontophoresis which is usually very effective, particularly for the hands, feet and armpits. In this treatment the affected body parts are held for about 20 minutes in a water bath through which a mild continuous electrical current is passed. In the case of the armpits, wet sponges are used. In a completely painless way, this method reduces the activity of the sweat glands. After two months it is possible to assess whether the therapy is working. Since perspiration is closely linked to the autonomic nervous system, there is a good chance that neurofeedback will significantly reduce excessive sweating.

Syncope
See Fainting fits

Teeth grinding (bruxism)
Jaw muscles are among the strongest muscles in the body, and so clenching or grinding the teeth at night can put an enormous stress on the skeleton. Whereas in normal chewing when the teeth meet the pressure exerted is 1-3 kilos, in bruxism the pressure is about 70 –80 kilos – and this is often sustained for hours. This is why in the long term this unconscious behavior can not only ruin the teeth but also give rise to many other problems such as tinnitus, chronic dizziness, migraine and trigeminal neuralgia (pain in the facial nerves near the jaw).

This happens particularly when the patient has problems arising from occlusion, i.e. when the upper and lower jaw do not come together as they should because of crooked teeth, badly fitting crowns and fillings or because the jawbone is out of line. Of course it is important to have such misalignments investigated but what is even more important is to eliminate the cause of clenching at night. Neurofeedback can help with this.
See also Stress

Tension headaches
This mild to moderate pain affects the whole head. There is a feeling of pressure and tautness in the head, sometimes the pain is also stabbing, but not throbbing. It is usually caused by tension resulting from stress which results in a headache either directly or via teeth grinding or a

body posture which is physiologically suboptimal. Neurofeedback can effectively relax both the inner tension and the tensed muscles and thus reduce the tendency to develop headaches.

Tics

Tics are uncontrolled bursts of certain movement and speech patterns, ranging from simple muscular twitches and constant clearing of the throat to inappropriate or even obscene utterances. This is due to a lack of impulse control. This can be highly effectively improved by neurofeedback training.

Tinnitus

For some people hearing noises for which there is no an external source is extremely distressing. There are very many causes, and these must be investigated before beginning neurofeedback treatment. Since there is usually (also) some impairment in the area of the cerebral cortex responsible for the processing of sound – the auditory cortex is overstimulated –, in many cases neurofeedback can alleviate tinnitus.

Tourette syndrome

People with this functional disturbance of the brain typically develop a whole range of tics (see Tics).

Trauma

See Post-traumatic stress disorder (PTSD)

Traumatic brain injury / craniocerebral trauma

See Brain damage

Traumatic stress reactions

Post-traumatic stress disorder / Traumatic stress reactions